Thirty Six Years in the NHS: My Nursing

VIVIEN OGDEN.

Dedication.

To my favourites.

Acknowledgments.

My grateful thanks to all who worked with me through the years. I emphasise that the views and opinions expressed in this book are purely personal, and based on my experience. I would also like to thank Jane Loftus for her help with this book

Introduction.

I have often said I ought to write a book, and now I have the time to do so. The process has been cathartic, I am amazed how much I remembered when I really thought about my career, and how much things have changed in the NHS. I hope it will be of interest to both those who have a nursing background, and those who do not. In view of this I have tried to make any medical terminology as clear as possible, and there is a glossary at the end of the book

Contents

Chapter 1: In The Beginning

So this is it, my last day of work ever!. I get out of bed, to put on my navy dress with the red piping round the collar for the last time. I pin the fob watch inside one of the lower pockets, and automatically add a couple of black pens. Then work routine of breakfast, and checking phone and emails. In the past ten weeks everyone has been given a lap top and mobile working has started. I contact IT (information technology) support as is often necessary, and end by thanking them for their help over the past few weeks, and explain this will be my last call. There is a slight pause, and the IT specialist says how good it is to have some thanks for the team, as it does not often happen

In ten minutes I am at my desk at the clinic where I am based just up the road. All is quiet, the time is eight o'clock and I aim to leave work at four pm. These hours stemmed from a time when the NHS had a work life balance initiative, and within reason hours were flexible, I held on to these hours. Everyone else does eight thirty to four thirty, a miniscule example of all the changes that have occurred over the past thirty six years.

My nurse training to be an SRN (state registered nurse) started in February 1978. I had not gained a place at the Radcliffe Infirmary in Oxford, as they felt I would not cope with the academic work. However with my mix of O level and GCSE qualifications I was accepted by the Royal Berkshire Hospital School of Nursing in Reading

On the appointed start day our set of about thirty students met for the first time in the sitting room of the nurses home in Craven Road (this is now the new main hospital entrance and a car park). Two matronly tutors, Miss R and Mrs V welcomed us to the hospital, explained the outline of the course and handed out our uniforms. This consisted of two white dresses, we were informed that for the first year there was no belt, then a blue belt in the second year, and black in the final year, providing the necessary exams and placements were passed. To be worn over the dress between wards or on night duty a dark navy wool cloak was issued, with a red lining, and fastenings that came over each shoulder, crossed over in front and fastened together with a button round the back.

Each of us also received a handful of thin white cardboard hats. These came with a little stud to hold them in shape once folded, and then needed hair grips to hold them on. They had superseded the cloth caps, and the cardboard ones were discontinued soon after my training. It was deemed they could be a safety hazard, they slipped easily and could catch in overhead bed rails, and it also saved money by getting rid of a useless piece of dress. Everyone had to purchase their own shoes, on inspection mine were unsuitable. The pre course list stated "flat brown shoes", apparently this meant lace up, and mine were slip on

Each student was then allocated a room; mine was at the end of the corridor on the top floor, with a shared bathroom and kitchen. In the second year students had the option to move out into student houses (these like the nurses home no longer exist). The rooms in the nurses home had a bed, wardrobe, bedside table and wash basin, and were very hot as there was little control over the radiator. We settled in, chatted and made friends. I was not there very much, boyfriends were of course not allowed, my fiancé, Alistair used to sneak in, along with various others seeing their girlfriends. The house mistresses did not make this easy, and male footprints on the floor were an obvious give away, and had to be hastily removed to avoid detection. Before I moved out the fire alarm went off one night. Everyone had to assemble outside; pandemonium ensued, caused by illicit occupants and the register being two years out of date, it took ages before we could get back to bed. I usually stayed with Alistair on his boat, and moved there in the August when we got married.

The training started with six weeks in The School of Nursing, on the hospital site next to the nurse's home. Compared with facilities provided for students in 2014 this was luxury. Nowadays students are university and not hospital based, and have a hectic life travelling the M4 corridor for lessons, tutorials and placements that stretch from London to Newbury, such is progress! Our initial learning was mainly biology, physiology, and nursing procedures in the practical room. Students were taught how to record temperature pulse and blood pressure. We used thermometers and syphgmonometers (blood pressure machines) that contained mercury, (since discontinued),and learnt bed bathing, temperature control with tepid sponging, catheter care, wound dressing, and bandaging. How to give suppositories, enemas, injections, and nasogastric care, thankfully we did not have to practice these skills on each other, just the former ones mentioned. I volunteered to be bed bathed, and was allowed to wear my bikini under the carefully folded red blanket, used specifically for bed baths. We joked anything could be hidden under a big red blanket, as this blanket would be frequently referred to by the tutors in practical work.

There was not the huge amount of academic work that students are expected to produce today, we had to produce an essay on a nursing topic for the end of the placement. For this we were shown how to use the nursing library. There were no computers, and all references had to be looked up in a reference catalogue, and then the appropriate journal or book located. This was very time consuming. The essays submitted were hand written and did not have to be referenced as they are today. Nursing was not the researched based profession it has become, and the information available was basic. Without computer search engine development, along with word processing, it would have been impossible to produce the quality and amount of academic work required by the university courses of today.

The time required to gather information however took just as long, and instead of online searches it was necessary to visit the library each time. On one of these many trips I decided that our old Ford Dexter tractor needed a run to charge the battery, and duly arrived at the School of Nursing where the library was situated. This caused quite a stir, as a tractor is not usually seen in a hospital car park. Several of the tutors came to see me off, they didn't know what to make of it, as I sprayed a liberal dose of Easystart into the air intake and the engine roared into life with a thick puff of smoke.

About two weeks into school we were taken on a ward visit in uniform. Not difficult as for some strange reason all students had to wear uniform every day in school. This would be the ward for the first ward based placement, mine was Adelaide ward. I had no idea what to expect, or really what a nurse did. There was no requirement to have experienced some sort of care work, as there is with today's training, and I was unknowingly a prime example of this necessity. My perception was that the doctor gave the orders and nurses carried them out, it hadn't crossed my mind that doctors were human, and as liable to make a mistake as anyone else. In some part this view was justified, as the push to get nursing recognised as a profession in its own right was in its infancy. I had chosen to go into nursing, purely because I enjoyed biology at school. Careers advice from school pleased that I had an idea of what I wanted to do had amounted to provision of nursing application contacts.

The early shift started at seven thirty in the morning. I gingerly let myself in, turning the brass doorknob of the large oak door that led off the imposing nineteenth century main hall and hospital entrance. The other side of the door to the left were two bays of four beds each, a couple of side rooms, the sluice and the laundry cupboard. On the other side was sister's office, the kitchen, store room and nurses cloak room. The corridor led onto the main high Nightingale ward, with bathrooms, toilets and more beds on the balcony at the far end. All the staff on duty congregated in sister's office for hand over from night to day staff. To me it was mind boggling to have name, age, diagnosis and brief update on thirty patients, all in half an hour as the night staff went off duty at eight am.

Sister on duty, allocated a fellow student in the year above for me to shadow, and handed out the duties for the morning written in the work book. The patients were listed by name and bed position/ number in this book, with their nursing requirements next to them. At the bottom of the page was a list of other jobs like laundry unpacking, sluice cleaning, restocking the back trolley and so on. The nurses worked in pairs and had between eight and ten patients, the length of time to attend to each patient was dependent on their level of need. Some were classed as "self caring ", so could wash themselves once given a wash bowl or taken to the bathroom.

I had not seen many adults in the nude, something I soon became used to as my buddy and I did bed baths, gave out bedpans, and neatly made the beds, mirroring each other's movements, as practised in school. The morning passed quickly, I couldn't understand why no one had been down for an operation yet. My buddy laughed and explained to me the difference between a surgical ward, where people needed surgery, and a medical ward where they were treated conservatively without operations, I was on a medical ward.

Adelaide ward had two sisters, as did most wards in 1978. Sister B was scary and old school, with beady black eyes, cloth cap and apron over her long sleeved navy dress with a stud collar, she did not miss a trick. Junior Sister G, a buxom motherly type, had a similar uniform except with short sleeves adorned with white caplets, both wore a black belt, and the silver buckle of a trained nurse. The other nurses of the ward team consisted of staff nurses (SN) in saxe blue, state enrolled nurses (SEN) in green, and auxiliary nurses in yellow, the cleaners wore a checked housecoat.

 Doctors were not on the ward all the time, and did rounds between the other medical wards. They had a long sleeved white coat over their own clothes, collar and tie for men and smart dress for ladies, a stethoscope was kept in one pocket, or in ready to use position round the neck, that is with the metal ear pieces either side of the neck. White coats are no longer used due to the long sleeves that prevented adequate hand washing, and the inability of some doctors to have them regularly laundered. The stethoscope has developed a new trendy position slung round the back of the neck if not in use.

That first eight week placement was an eye opener, and a good grounding for what was to come. There was plenty of hands on experience, students were salaried, and counted in the ward staff numbers, today students have a bursary, and are supernúmery to ward staff. So our input was really needed and the sooner skills learnt in school could be transferred to the ward the better. It would be later in my training that the Nursing Process came into use, so the work tended to be task rather than patient orientated. For example two nurses would do a back round of everyone on the ward, to prevent or treat pressure sores. A large trolley laid up with clean sheets, nighties, pyjamas, wash bowel, soap, paper wipes, and a variety of agents thought to be beneficial to pressure sores or their prevention. Methylated spirits or talc was vigorously rubbed on unbroken bottoms, elbows, heels etc, and honey, egg white and oxygen or cod liver oil cream applied to broken areas often with no dressing, this practice went out as there was no research to back them, other than to show them ineffective, or harmful.

The back round for high dependency patients occurred every two hours, this number had stemmed from the amount of time it took at Stoke Mandeville Burns Unit, to get round all the patients and start again. Positioning patients and changing them was hard work, sometimes we had just finished and the person was incontinent again, or could not be got in a comfortable position. In among this was the constant requests for bed pans, bed pan rounds were made, but the patients couldn't always oblige at the allotted time.

My first injection given to a patient was on Adelaide ward, a hydroxocobalamine (VitaminB12), for iron deficiency anaemia. The drug came as a clear red liquid in a small glass ampoule. The Staff Nurse and I carefully checked the ampoule against the prescription details on the medicine chart, difficult to see as written in black against dark red. Then I put the two ml plastic syringe together with a blue needle, the correct one for the type and site of injection to be given. Opening the ampoule required a knack, and care had to be taken not to cut yourself, and drawing up the liquid I was all fingers and thumbs. We proceeded to the patient, checked the name of the person by asking their name, and looked at their wrist band.

Then, the moment of truth. I puckered up the skin and

muscle on the upper arm, and introduced the needle. The person was very thin, perhaps not the best candidate for a first injection, and there was a sudden stop as the needle hit the bone, the staff nurse saw my face, calmly advised to withdraw the needle slightly, and carry on. She explained after that the patient would be unlikely to notice, and a bone touch was of more concern to the nurse. Everyone was under strict instruction not to re-sheath the needle, as this could result in a needle stick injury. The needle complete with syringe should be placed straight into the sharps box. A sharps box, made of thick grease proof cardboard, came flat and a nursing task was to make them up for use. It was not uncommon for a used needle to poke through, so a tough yellow plastic container later replaced the cardboard version.

On one shift I was asked to go over to Sidmouth Ward. To my surprise when I got there I knew Sister W who was on duty, it was a real turn of the tables. I had trained as a BHSAI (British Horse Society Assistant Instructor), while I waited to start my nurse training. Sister W had been one of my pupils at Wellington Riding, in the Saturday afternoon reasonable rider adult class. As the riders went round I would give commands, to correct position of horse and rider."Jerry, get your weight into your heels, prepare for canter at the corner, and canter NOW..". We both looked at each other in complete surprise, we chatted about horses for a short while, and then nursing etiquette resumed. Sister W lived with another women, and was a source of fascinating speculation to the working pupils at Wellington Riding.

Breathlessness due to various causes, occurred frequently on the ward, and a common part of emergency admission treatment would be Friar's Balsam via a Nelson inhaler. The inhaler, made of china with "Nelson Inhaler" on it was crazed and years old. Hot water poured over a teaspoon of Friar's Balsam mixed the inhalation, the mouthpiece, made of glass had a piece of gauze wrapped round it, through which the patient inhaled. Health and Safety, with boiling water, glass between teeth, and inability to properly clean the drop shape vessel, saw the end of this inhalation

Death of a person is an inevitable experience for a student, and will happen somewhere in training, it is unusual to qualify and not have been involved in the care of a dying person. My first death was on my first ward, I had gleaned by then that not everyone got well and went home, and was not quite sure what happened. This particular patient was very cachexic with terminal lung cancer. She was really breathless and very thin, the effort of breathing was clearly visible as the intercostal spaces rose and fell between the ribs, and her shoulders heaved up and down. With childhood asthma, and poor initial treatment, I had some experience of what being short of breath meant, and had come across nothing like this before. Everything from washing, feeding, drinking, and all activities of daily living required help. The nasal cannulae poked into her nose and made it sore, I applied Vaseline to the skin which eased her discomfort. She constantly needed to be sat bolt upright in bed, the most comfortable position, and despite a pillow rolled in a draw sheet, and tucked tightly over the mattress, down the patient slid. I had heard about Cheyenne Stoke breathing as the body shuts down to death, and sure enough the breathing pattern became uneven, and secretions rattled in the chest. There were prolonged gaps with no breath, until I thought the lady had gone, and went to pull the sheet up over her face, when she took another gasp, so I folded the sheet down. The situation was quite frightening, and I had to disturb Sister B on the drug round to come and see the patient, Sister B agreed death was imminent and carried on with the drugs. I sat with the lady who slipped away.

Chapter 2:Placements at Battle and RBH

Each ward placement was six to eight weeks long, with around six weeks in school each year. At the time Battle Hospital on the Oxford Road was open, and at least half the placements were there. The original part of the hospital had been a work house, where currently geriatric, orthopaedic and casualty were crammed into old outdated wards. There was major debate as to whether RBH and Battle should be combined, and if so on which site, or should a new hospital be built outside Reading at Swallowfield? The pros and cons of each site were debated at length, the decision fell to finance as it often does. The RBH became the main hospital, as a lot of money had been spent there, the Maternity Unit, Eye Block, and South Wing already complete, and the expense of discarding these facilities could not be justified.

A new cook chill food facility was built at Battle; I think to replace hospital kitchens on both sites. For one reason or another the completed building with all the catering equipment was never used, and eventually demolished, a criminal waste of public money. The new RBH transformed the site, with the demolition of the old Elm House in the middle, to what is now the new link corridor, wards on three levels and the multi-story car park where the Nurses Home once stood. The wards in the old part of the hospital on the London Road have been updated as far as is possible within the constraint of the building, and eventually may not be used as wards at all.

Five of my placements were at Battle. Tilehurst Ward, the far end of the one story sixties building was surgical. Sister H was a stickler for fluid charts; the amount a patient took in and put out over twenty four hours, one subtracted from the other and a total obtained for that period. At the time it seemed laborious, with hindsight she definitely had a point.

Part of nurse training meant four practical assessments had to be passed. For some reason I chose to do my drug assessment on the paediatric ward, paediatric doses are all different and smaller than the adult dose. The assessment took place on a drug round where every aspect had to be correct, from management of the trolley, e.g. locking it if called away, double checking the identity of the patient, and that the prescription was correct. Hence the importance of knowing the correct dose of each drug, side effects and interaction, sensitivity and so on. On the prescription sheet the time and dose for each drug was recorded, and a note made if more needed to be ordered from pharmacy. There seemed so many drugs to learn, and things changed all the time, for me it has always been one of the most difficult aspects of nursing, as there is no room for error. I was thankful to pass and move on, I did not really enjoy nursing children, the parents would do the caring, so the duty dragged, unless an emergency happened then everything was frantic.

Chiltern Ward in the old part of the hospital was an upstairs Nightingale style ward, on the face of it old and shabby. However to me, drawn to historic relics, the ward had several Interesting features. One loo had the old high cistern on intricate iron brackets, with an ornate china handle on the end of a chain inscribed PULL. The toilet bowl, an early Armitage Shanks, china crazed, with a wooden seat (no lid). The basins were of the same vintage and there were substantial early radiators. The mantle- piece over the fireplace in the main ward was present, though the fireplace was blocked off. In the kitchen, a huge solid kitchen table with draws, and an antique six burner gas cooker built to last for ever. On the top rested a five pint kettle, and some other equally large utensils. The Ward Orderly lectured me on making the tea, as I had boiled the water and not immediately added it to the gigantic teapot that should have been warmed. According to her the tea would turn green.

On the ward many of the patients had been there for years, as there disabilities meant they could not look after themselves. This method of looking after geriatrics as they were known, changed during my training. People who had a stable condition, e.g. post stroke, now had a social as opposed to a medical need. The plan to move them all out to Nursing Home or Residential facilities was cutting edge and controversial. Now it is normal, and safer for patients as they do not languish in hospital unnecessarily. Sister on the ward who was grossly overweight, reminded me of a large spider scuttling down the short corridor to the office where she spent a considerable amount of time. I remember my draw dropped, as Sister said to a lady equal in size "I don't know how you manage to get yourself into this state..." turned and went for her next ample meal or snack in the kitchen.

Nurse training included a theatre placement. Orthopaedic theatre in the old part of Battle Hospital was run by Charge Nurse Mr P. Mr P, coming up for retirement, lived at home with his elderly mother, and had run the three theatres for years. He knew the three Surgeons very well, and had the knack of anticipating their every need. The first thing Mr P checked with a new student was hand washing technique, once satisfied the technique was correct , I was shown how to manage sterile and non sterile areas in theatre. To start with this would be standing watching, and not touching anything. It felt special as instead of uniform everyone wore scrubs, and white clogs. Operations could be anything from carpel tunnel repair, to emergency burr hole for pressure brain injury. Under supervision I could suture in minor surgery, and so passed my wound care assessment, where asepsis is paramount. Several afternoons a week were devoted to planned hip surgery, a cheerful event that involved a lot of sawing and banging as the trochanter was prepared and the new prosthetic hip inserted. Mr C was the senior Surgeon, one op he looked at me over the top of his mask, and asked for what I thought was an egg timer. I scoured the shelves to no avail, it turned out he was after size eight gloves.

The surgical team medics changed frequently as they under went their own development. A new Registrar, Mr D caused quite a stir. On his first day I helped him with his operating gown. The gowns had a paper tape attached to the tie of the gown. To maintain sterility the surgeon put on his gown, handed the tape to the un-scrubbed nurse, who held it so he could do a full body twirl so the ties could be secured in front, without reaching behind. Once facing the nurse again a string taken in each gloved hand, a nod would signal to the nurse to pull away the paper end, thus preserving the no touch technique. Mr D seemed to have no idea how to do this. In theatre with the other surgeons he seemed hesitant and relied on the scrubbed nurse for the correct instrument. About a week later he disappeared from the team. Sister on the orthopaedic ward had become suspicious at the new Registrar's interest in the controlled drugs cupboard, and had found a discrepancy in the stock control. It turned out Mr D was a drug addict impostor. Under a false name he had managed to wangle his way through the interview, and must have had false references, or they had not been checked. Thankfully in the induction period, he did not get his hands on a scalpel.

On the weekend in theatre only emergency surgery

happened. There might be periods with not much going on, so everyone did deep cleaning and checked all the equipment. This entailed taking all the stores out of the high glass fronted cupboards, checking the package condition and expiry date, and washing the shelves. The main Honeywell theatre, a clever instant theatre designed by an American company had been a competitively priced option to update the old theatre. The hexagonal domed pod in pale blue came complete with air tight doors, internal shelves, operating lights and table, and was easily erected in any space large enough. From the outside it looked like something from NASA as it sat in the old theatre. It was past its best, and needed running repairs to keep it going. Mr P had his own workshop within the building, a happy hour meant helping him. One of the jobs was to repair the theatre light bulb with plaster of Paris, as he said they were far too expensive to replace. Under the operating table the old ripped lino required attention with various tapes and glue. Today this type of equipment service would not be covered by vicarious insurance (and probably would not have been back then).

Ward management assessment tended to be towards the end of training as it tested the ability to run all aspects of ward nursing and administration for a shift. Castle ward at Battle, in the same block as Tilehurst Ward, had respiratory patients, most of whom came in as an emergency. They would be breathless, frightened and required immediate nursing and medical treatment. Sister who was very competent, smoked like a chimney, and boasted a peak flow of 500 lpm (litres per minute) a good reading of which she was very proud. The fact that most of the patients admitted had smoking related illness did not bother her. Anyway, the assessment started with taking handover from the night staff at the beginning of my shift. Change in patient condition, care and new patients were all discussed in turn, and I allocated the morning work. After checking the crash trolley, and doing the medicine round, patient round with sister and then the doctors followed. I had to know a fair amount about every patient, and then from my list made on the rounds, organise specimens, investigations, porters, order pharmacy and ward stock etc. Frequent interruption is inevitable on a busy ward, so it was necessary to be able to prioritise, and reorganise as required. The shift flew by and sister sat down with me to discuss the day, I had managed pretty well on a very busy shift, and apart from a couple of minor things I can't remember, I was fine.

Chapter 3: Nursing Night and Day.

As a student we did a fair amount of night duty, eight nights on and six off, which changed to seven on, seven off later on. In effect the time off was reduced as the first day off after working all night was a wash-out, and before going back on duty after nights off, I had a restful day. I ended up doing twenty weeks over the time I trained. The shift started at nine pm and finished at eight am with a half hour overlap each end for handover. After handover the patients would be settled for the night, late drug round made, and lights out. Sometimes the night could be really busy. With a skeleton staff we dealt with patients who were very poorly, post operation, and new admissions if the ward was on take. Early in my second year I started holding the ward keys: that meant you were in charge. Though this practice has gone, and students are no longer expected to be in charge so early in training, it was common when I trained, and certainly provided plenty of experience of ward management.

The hospital was run by two night sisters, or a sister and number 7 (known previously, and now, as matron). They did their rounds of all the wards before midnight, and could be bleeped if required at any time. On the ward round it would be expected that I knew all the details of up to thirty patients by heart. This was difficult as there was a great deal to remember. One night frantically trying to recall some patient details, sister said "I am sure you said he had a hemi colectomy, not a hernia repair", when I looked it up later, he had had a hernia repair, phew!

Trained staff were not immune from mistakes, one busy night on Chiltern Ward at Battle there were two patients imminently near to death, and the first died. Night Sister rang the relative of the other patient. This meant she had the awful task of phoning to say she had made a mistake. Then the person did die, and necessitated yet another call. Poor sister was shattered and miserable by the end of the night. Night duty is shattering, one morning I pulled up on my Honda 70, my transport at the time, and sat at the hospital entrance ready to turn left on to the Oxford road. In my tired state my eyes were glued to the red man on the pedestrian crossing light on my left. As soon as it turned to the green man I pulled out, nearly winging a pedestrian who also responded to the green man!

If the night was quiet on Victoria Ward the staff sat one either end as the ward was separated by the office and sluice. Reading anything other than a nursing journal or text book was not allowed, and no drink on the desk. The night could drag, and we would cough discreetly to the nurse in the other end if Sister approached, so offending items could be hidden. At break time which usually happened after midnight the canteen was open so you could go for a meal. If the night was quiet we used to extend our breaks to a couple of hours each, this meant time for a sleep. The linen cupboard or office made up with a pillow and blankets could be very cosy, frowned upon of course, though common practice. The problem was waking up afterwards, I would sit with a hot drink praying nothing would need doing before I had properly come too.

One night on Nuffield Ward there had been barely time for a break at all, I was on with SN PT. PT, was a very overbearing person, who bossed me about all night. Near the end of the shift an emergency admission arrived who needed to be admitted, catheterised and a nasogastric tube passed. By the time I had done all this I was late home, and missed seeing my husband before he left for work. This low point tempted me to give up nursing altogether. Years later I nursed PT in the community, she had become a lonely anxious old lady. She didn't recognise me in my now more senior role to hers, and her over bearing manor no longer bothered me.

I was on duty on Christmas night in the second year of my training, and I remember all the sisters wore their cloaks inside out so the red lining showed, which gave a very festive air to the night. I had my long striped socks on, and sister felt she had to draw the line at that, so I took them off. At break time around midnight, everyone was invited down in turn for Christmas dinner, turkey with all the trimmings, Christmas pudding, and even a small glass of wine. Back then alcohol at work was acceptable in moderation, and each ward had a table full of chocolates and beverages for staff to help themselves. The night sisters had decorated the canteen, and served the meal to all the staff, after which we waddled back to our wards.

On duty on Victoria a general surgical ward, I frequently undertook the care and maintenance of a patient's colostomy. I had never heard of a colostomy before I started nursing. In training we were taught about them, the reason they were needed, and how to look after them. Protective gloves were not to be worn, as it would embarrass the patient and make them feel dirty. On the ward staff debated this, as no one wanted to handle someone else's faeces, and they all wore gloves, the staff rightly pointed out gloves protected the nurse form contamination. Gloves soon became obligatory and part of hospital infection control policy. A clean colostomy bag had to replace the used bag each day, it was a smelly affair for everyone, and I soon got the hang of the quick change

Sometimes, particularly post op the bag would burst, the poor patient could be covered, literally from head to toe, a full wash and change of all bedding would take two of us about half an hour. There were various air fresheners to mask the smell, none of which worked much. A loop colostomy is raised in an emergency obstruction of the bowel, and once the obstruction is resolved the temporary colostomy would be re-sectioned with the bowel and abdomen sewn up. The distal end of the bowel had to be washed out in preparation for theatre. This could be a messy affair, one afternoon the patient and I decided to try tackling the procedure in the bathroom. Gently inserting the rubber tube and liquid into the bowel I thought we were well prepared with numerous paper incontinence sheets. Despite this we both ended up paddling in the un- mentionable. Staff nurse poked her head round the door in response to the laughter, to see student nurse and patient had seen the funny side to the situation.

The bowel theme is integral throughout nursing, everyday on every ward I worked on, each patient would be asked about their bowels on the morning round. If the answer was "no" three days running, time for intervention. This would mean giving suppositories, and if this was not effective, an enema. Green enema saponis (soap) mixed with warm water in a plastic jug was introduced into the rectum via a disposable rectal catheter, connected to an orange rubber tube and funnel. The patient lay on their left side while the liquid flowed in, and had to make a hasty retreat to the commode ready at the bedside. The enema kit of rubber tube and funnel, was then sent back to CSSD (Central Sterile Supply Department) in a yellow plastic bag, to be re-sterilised and issued back to the ward for next time. The use of enema saponis went out, as there were too many risks, and needless discomfort for the patient. Now constipation is mainly treated with modern laxatives, and suppositories or a five millilitre micro enema if required.

To continue with the bowel, if a patient had excess flatus that they were unable to pass, a flatus tube inserted into the rectum bought relief, or so it was believed in the late seventies. A disposable rectal catheter was used, and the end held under water in a kidney dish and evidence of flatus seen as bubbles. No proof of effectiveness backed the procedure, flatus will find its own way out, and the occasional male patient derived sexual pleasure from it, not the aim of the procedure. The vulval douche performed on obstetric wards, where the pregnant lady sat in bed on a bed pan, and the nurse poured warm chlorhexidine in water over the vulval area, has also been discontinued for the same reason. Embarrassing for patient and nurse, these ladies were capable of their own hygiene needs

Chapter 4: Scary Placement and I Deliver a Baby.

At the end of our second year, we had a choice of a three month placement in community health or obstetrics. Everyone received a taster of the placement not chosen. For me this meant a day at Borough Court, a severe educationally subnormal unit, and a day at the mental health facility, Fairmile Hospital. At Borough Court I found the patients alarming, and had difficulty discerning patients from staff, as no one wore uniform, I cowered behind the entrance door. The building compounded the scene. Borough Court, built by a rich industrialist in flamboyant gothic style, boasted a huge oak front door, and a grand staircase with stained glass windows. In the main hall ornate gas lamps (electrified) lit the way along the passage of red brick gothic arches. The light from the lamps threw shadows on the ornate tiled floor, and the odd scream or shout in the distance echoed along the corridor. The house had a second narrow staircase that led to the sparse servant quarters in the attic under the eves of the steeply pointed roof. The rooms had recently had patients in them, but had been converted to store rooms. As no one seemed particularly interested in a student nurse, I explored the house

Fairmile Hospital at South Stoke had been specially built as a mental institution in the late eighteen hundreds. I arrived for my day, and met up with staff nurse as directed. He explained that they treated a broad range of mental health problems, schizophrenia, paranoia, depression, acute suicidal patients and so on. The George Schuster Unit, a prefab in the grounds, was a locked ward and held patients who as a danger to themselves or the public, needed to be detained. When the hospital opened these people would have been locked in the individual cells, which staff nurse showed me in the main building. These cells were the same as those in a prison, sparse, no window and heavy locked door. Other unfortunates would be kept prone in a metal cage, and a variety of dubious, supposedly curative treatments given

Electro convulsive therapy (ECT), invented to help with severe depression among other diagnoses is still used today. The original ECT theatre was a museum, with a newer facility close by. The procedure is now conducted with the use of muscle relaxants; this made the procedure more humane, and avoided horrendous muscle contraction. There was talk of Fairmile being closed in the future, and the inmates of many years moved into the community. One of these people had originally been admitted to Fairmile for having a child out of wedlock, and another the village idiot. Years of ineptitude and institulisation had rendered Fairmile home, and the prospect of moving into sheltered housing must have been frightening. Smoking, once considered a beneficial medical treatment still appeared very much in evidence as staff and I walked round the red brick hospital. Each ward had high ceilings and windows, through a haze of cigarette smoke patients and staff sat puffing away, seated in chairs round the edge of the room. Despite it being late morning most patients wore their striped pyjamas. Staff nurse explained that the smoking kept the patients calm. The smoke combined with a strong smell of wee, made my eyes water.

These two placements compounded that mental and physical disability nursing were not for me. Both Fairmile and Borough Court are now luxury apartments, and the previous inhabitants settled in smaller family orientated houses, or purpose built facilities in the community. Those that require acute intervention are admitted to the new Prospect Park Hospital, and discharged home as soon as possible.

All the maternity and obstetric wards were in a purpose built facility on the Craven Road side of the RBH. On the top floor the special care baby unit, convenient to maternity, and a gynae ward. I started on the obstetric ward, where pre term ladies were admitted. They came to this ward if there was a problem with the pregnancy, such as high blood pressure, bleeding, or reduced foetal movement. Though some of the patients were on bed rest for threatened abortion, everyone was able to look after themselves, as far as hygiene was concerned. Unfortunately spontaneous abortion occasionally became inevitable, and the lady would be moved to a side room while nature took its course. This showed me how painful, both physically and emotionally abortion was, and the special type of support required. On my gynae ward experience there had been planned abortions, and some women appeared to use it as a method of contraception. Despite this and what ever the reason for abortion emotional support, making life as comfortable as possible proved a large part of nursing these ladies. The pathetic little foetus lying in a kidney dish in the sluice, was a sobering end to a life and a shift. On ethical/ religious grounds, we were told we did not have to take part in planned abortion, I had neither objection, and most of the other students also nursed these women, and teenagers.

Special care Baby Unit, or SCBU as it was always called, resided on the top floor of the Maternity Building, up four flights of stairs. I preferred to run up the stairs instead of taking the lift as an easy way to fit in some exercise in the day. The gym never has been, or will be a place for me. Why spend money on exercise when it can be free at work, or for that matter free and beneficial at home?. If I cleaned the car or mowed the lawn, I exercised, had the satisfaction of a job completed, and neither paid gym membership or someone else to do my chores, a win win situation all round for me.

SCBU where I went for some of my obstetric placement was always terribly busy, and often fraught with emotion. The tiny babies needed so much care and thought, and doctors, nurses and parents would have to make difficult treatment decisions on a daily basis, I admired all the staff who worked there. A few of the babies had conditions such as hair lip and cleft pallet, and needed skill and patience to feed via nasogastric tube, or custom made plastic upper pallet inserts to help them suck until they had reconstructive surgery. Other congenital abnormalities would require a lifetime of care, and I admired the parents that were at the beginning of a long path of devotion to a child who would remain a child in an adult body. If one of these babies died, plenty of time to say goodbye would be made for the grieving parents, who grieved for their loss, yet also realised it was arguably the best outcome for a severely disabled baby. Of course the majority of babies were just born early, and with care and attention went home and caught up with their peers, and no one would ever guess how they had clung to life in their first weeks of life.

The Maternity Suite was the hub of operations, and central to the placement. As part of admission ladies who came to the ward in labour would routinely have the vulval area shaved, and be given two suppositories to clear the bowel. Both procedures since discontinued. They would then be settled in to a delivery room, and could be almost ready to give birth, or spend hours in labour. Along with the midwife I would monitor. This included abdominal palpation to determine the baby's position, watching the heart monitor for a drop in heart beat, maternal blood pressure, noting when the waters broke, number, strength and frequency of contractions and so on. I did not do vaginal examination to determine cervical dilatation, this was performed by the midwife. Back then as a student I was able to deliver three babies. The midwife and I would scrub up together, and she would guide my hand to steady the rate of delivery and reduce perineal tares, as the crown of the babies head came into view. Nerve racking and a relief when the body followed, and baby could be united with mum. In the excitement and trauma of birth, the ladies seldom noticed an episiotomy cut, or injection for uterine contraction, and delivery of the placenta. After cutting the umbilical cord, we were taught how to check the placenta and confirm condition. The placentas were frozen, and sent off to, I think a beauty product firm.

At the end of the placement I received my Obstetric Certificate with practical and theory passed. I enjoyed the placement, but for me it seemed repetitive, and a career as a midwife? Probably not

Chapter 5: Oncology Orthopaedics and Casualty

West ward in the old part of the hospital, had Sister G in charge of the oncology (cancer) ward, for in patients that needed palliative radio or chemotherapy. People were often very poorly when admitted, and quite a few died. One evening a lady came in, and Sister asked me to admit her. To my surprise Mrs L had been my baby sitter. Mum would get her to come round, and sometimes bring her husband Charlie. Charlie mortified us three children by singing along with the Henley Symphony Orchestra, when everyone else silently listened. At the age of fourteen I pointed out to Mum that my friends were baby sitting themselves, so the Ls stopped coming. Mrs L had a great deal of back pain, and it was difficult to make her comfortable. She had ignored her own deterioration in health, determined to look after Charlie who being epileptic had frequent fits. Despite her own pain she nursed him to the end, before going to the doctor herself. She died later that evening, at least Mrs L knew me, as there was no family.

Sister G was old school, and still wore a long sleeve dress and cloth cap. She had piercing dark eyes, and whizzed round the ward like a sparrow, in her flat laced duty shoes. Gliding about it was difficult to tell where she would appear next. Her voice was very soft, and spoken quickly with a Scottish accent could be difficult to understand. After a second or third muttered reply when asked to repeat what was said, it would be down to guess work as to the nature of the request. As a student I did not feel I could ask yet another time as to what she wanted. Despite this short coming I remember her as being very fair, and keen to involve the students with different patient conditions. All staff on the ward had a small blue plastic gygercounter, pinned to their uniform, to ensure no one received excess radio activity from patient treatment. If a lady had cancer of the cervix (neck of the womb), radio active rods would be inserted into the cervix in theatre. For ten days, the person, nursed in a side room, had staff access for essentials only. The gygercounters were checked at the end of her treatment for the staff involved. No outcome as to the radio therapy risk was given to students, so I guess the level remained safe.

Before supper on a late shift, the patients were offered an alcoholic beverage. Sister explained that despite possible medication interaction, this medicament helped the soul, and improved appetite, especially sherry. The drinks trolley had everything from spirits to wine and beer, with accompanying tonic, lemonade, ice, sliced lemon, etc, the glasses that tinkled together didn't match, and some were cut glass. If a person's fancy did not appear on the trolley, this would be purchased out of ward funds. The patients enjoyed their drinks, and it gave a cosy home feel to the day.

As training progressed students were allowed to

perform female urinary catheterisation, (male catheterisation performed by doctors only, or occasionally an experienced male nurse).This procedure required a certain technique, and to maintain sterility good skill and dexterity. In the younger female the urethra is easy to see when the labia are parted, and the tip of the catheter inserted without touching any surrounding part. However in more elderly ladies the anatomy changes due to menopause, and the urethra retracts out of sight. I had seen catheterisation performed, and assembled the equipment on the trolley, a CSSD pack, latex catheter the right size etc. (Latex is now always coated with hydrogel or made of silicon as people can be allergic to latex). Under the watchful eye of staff nurse I prepared the patient, and commenced the procedure.

That particular patient, though elderly was thin, so reasonably easy to catheterise, except her legs kept sliding out of position. The opportunity arose several times for me to catheterise. Some were very awkward and needed two as we burrowed in the fat folds of an obese patient, with a torch. First of all to get the legs positioned, and then to identify the appropriate anatomy, three or four catheters might be used as we struggled to maintain sterility.

The catheter, connected to a urine drainage bag hung on a stand at the side of the bed, the wire frames easily caught under the bed when it was lowered, so were a funny squashed shape. Catheter bags had to be emptied and measured regularly, and kept patent as a closed system to prevent infection. Catheter care consisted of a CSSD pack with galley pot and five cotton wool balls. These were dipped in sterile chlorhexidine, and wiped round the meatus where the catheter entered body. Research showed this increased the infection risk, and the procedure was replaced in favour of a good wash all round.

The amount of restraint that could or could not be used on a patient used to be more of a grey area than now, and of course is sometimes required if a patient is a danger to themselves or anyone else. Because of the uncertainty this could range from porters asked to physically restrain someone, to letting the person have free rein. On the medical ward Huntley and Palmer, that specialised in renal patients, I saw examples of both. In my naivety it was difficult to know, or decide what was acceptable, and looking back I think in general staff struggled with the problem, as there were no clear guidelines.

One gentleman who had gross oedema in limbs and trunk kept getting out of bed and falling, cot sides, draw sheets and close observation were of no avail, and he had to be manhandled back to bed protesting loudly. In contrast a very confused patient announced he wanted to leave, and the doctors and nurses said they were not allowed to restrain him. He duly left in his hospital gown, and spent two nights on a railway embankment before someone brought him back, cold dirty and hungry. It horrified me at the time; guidelines have since helped to manage these types of situations much better.

Towards the end of my training I had placements on Hunter Ward, trauma orthopaedics, and casualty, (now known as accident and emergency). All the orthopaedic wards, trauma and planned surgery had moved over from Battle while I trained, to the new and purpose built South Wing. Hunter Ward had thirty-two beds, consisting of four bays of six beds, and opposite, one four bedded bay, sluice and four side rooms, two behind the nurses station, and a small kitchen. A linen cupboard, dressing trolley room, a bathroom and toilets completed the ward layout. The ward sister and I got on with each other well from the start, she being a no nonsense Taurian like myself. With her black hair scraped into a high bun, pencilled eyebrows, and not quite regulation court shoes, fools were not suffered gladly, patients came first and that was that. With a haughty stare any doctor could be put in his place, yet the three consultants respected and trusted her.

Sister D had trained at the John Radcliffe, and frequently had us all in fits of laughter when she talked about some of the antics. At one time Sister and her fellow students decided going to bed was a waste of time, and stayed up for several days and nights in a row. Their strategy came to light when they were found to be fast asleep on duty, in the ward linen cupboard. They were all in big trouble and narrowly avoided being thrown out. Despite this misdemeanour Sister had passed her course, staffed on orthopaedics, and had worked on Kennet at Battle, moving to Hunter when the old ward closed.

The other members of the team consisted of Sister B the junior sister, a senior SN, four or five SNs , three SENs (state enrolled nurses), and Cath S the NA (Nursing Auxiliary). Between them there was years of experience, though not necessarily progression, and everyone got on well. Junior Sister could get in a flap and have everyone running around like mad, and the NA seemed to me to have as much knowledge as anyone else. Cath had a thing about seeing red and white flowers together, she would nearly go berserk as she said some one was about to die. The offending bunches would be whipped into the sluice for the addition of other colours. Flowers were allowed in those days, and a fair amount of time seemed to be spent attending to them. Why this should fall to the nurses is one I often pondered. On top of patient flowers, there would be ones donated from a funeral, so the ward would look like a flower shop, and make nursing difficult with the extra pots on each locker. The pots were pastel shades and light aluminium, battered and well used they wobbled and upset easily.

Each shift on a Hunter went quickly as there was so much happening. Sister D was a riot, and such fun to work with. Her attitude was that just because she was

Sister, there was no reason why she wouldn't work with her staff and students. I loved working with Sister D for a morning, the patients liked her bright cheery manor, and there would be lots to learn as you went. Lifting and handling technique, in it's infancy meant we used an Australian lift to move a patient of twenty fives stone up the bed. This entailed linking hands under the patient's thighs, putting our shoulders under the patient's haunch, and lifting on your other arms braced on the bed, knees bent and shifting weight from one foot to the other. This lift between two, was the accepted way to move a person up the bed. Later the Australian lift came under the spot light of health and safety at work, as a major cause of staff back injury. It carried immeasurable cost in both finance and time off sick, and is now forbidden. When I trained we thought nothing of lifting, and sister and I would extract ourselves from under the patient red faced from exertion, and laughing, on to the next. However there was a lift for the bath. The Ambulift could be fitted with a bath seat or a sling and wound up and down manually, this early lift heralded the beginning of the sophisticated hoists now available, and the move away from manual lifting of patients.

At the end of the morning we tidied the ward and got ready for the lunch trolley to be bought up from the kitchen. The full sacks of linen in the sluice, were tied up and put outside the ward for the laundry porter to collect, red for soiled and white bags for unsoiled.

Both metal back trolleys would be cleaned and replenished.

Our bete-noire proved to be the bedpan machine. The blue plastic bedpan shells, given out with a grey papier-mâché lining, once used and covered with a grey card lid, had to be put in the macerator. This fickle machine sprang into action once the lid was firmly closed, and the red button pushed. It jammed easily, if more than three pans were put in at once, or the grey tops, paper towels, or anything other than pan contents and loo roll entered the device. Sometimes it stopped for no apparent reason with the warning light on. So phone the engineer, and in the meantime the pans would pile up in miserable smelly heaps until he arrived to mend it, not a job I envied. The rest of the hospital had metal bedpans that got cleaned one at a time in a steamer operated by a handle and foot pedal. On Adelaide ward the last remaining bedpan boiler resided. About ten pans covered in water would be boiled, and hooked out with bed pan tongs to cool on a rack. Men's urinals on South Wing, also papier-mâché went in the masher, and glass urinals elsewhere cleaned with a pressure jet of water that went everywhere if it inadvertently got pressed with no bottle over it.

Casualty, my chosen final placement followed on from trauma orthopaedics. The pace usually did not let up all shift, with a packed waiting room. Students were allowed to do various procedures once observed by trained staff. A patient, who came in with a nail injury for example a thumb that had been shut in a door, would need the nail trephining, where a small puncture wound made in the nail would relieve the pressure underneath, and the pain. The best tool to do this would be a paper clip unbent, and one end stuck into a cork as a handle. The end, heated over a meths burner was then inserted through the nail, and the blood would spurt out in style all over the place, taking away the momentary discomfort of the paper clip passing through the nail. A very satisfying procedure to perform. Trauma wounds came in all shapes and sizes. If a wound had gravel embedded, a sterile soft scrubbing brush (nail brush size) in a pack with poverdine iodine would be used to remove the gravel, and forceps to painstakingly pick shards of glass out. I could soon tell which wounds needed to be sutured by the trained staff, or steri-stripped by me. Very useful to me as it is common for friends family etc to assume nurses know everything about wounds.

The patients seen came in with all sorts of afflictions. The trained staff soon let a patient know if they felt they were wasting time in casualty. A postman, who had been bitten on a testicle during his round, came under sister's wrath. Sister asked me to investigate, and though there was a bite, it only amounted to a tiny graze, with no sign of swelling or infection. He was sent packing with a comment to the effect of surely he didn't think this wound would need hospital intervention

Drug overdose was commonplace, various analgesics or an antidepressant taken with alcohol would be a usual cocktail that needed a gastric lavage (stomach pump). This fell to SEN Betty who had been on the unit for years, and would attack the patient who would be very low in mood, with her no nonsense skilled routine. The patient would be asked to swallow the nasogastric tube fitted to a funnel, inverted over a bucket to empty the contents of the stomach. The passing of the nasogastric gastric tube caused the patient to wretch and vomit, effective and unpleasant for all. Some patients would be regular visitors for gastric lavage, and appeared immune to the discomfort of the procedure. Invariably there would be follow up by the psychiatrist after a suicide attempt.

The psychiatrist also saw a patient for anything else that could be deemed mental as opposed to physical health. One young woman frequently came to Casualty with attention seeking behaviour, I specialed her in a side room on a shift, she became inconsolable, grabbed a flower vase and emptied the entire contents over her head. I didn't know what to do and felt completely helpless. One of the casualty sisters could distinguish between genuine anguish and a panic attack. A teenage girl I tried to reason with got more and more beside herself, crying and sobbing. Sister heard her, came in and told her to stop and pull herself together, which she promptly did. I asked sister about this intuition; she said it came with dealing with many similar situations.

Emergency admission of a person who had collapsed is known as a crash call. On route the ambulance crew would radio the department, as they blue lighted the patient to hospital. The crash (resuscitation) team in casualty, with doctors, anaesthetist, and nurses assembled to receive the patient, as speed is the essence in life saving treatment. In the resuscitation room all the equipment and drugs, checked and ready we waited for the patient. As a student I always had supervision in this scenario, and on this particular crash call staff nurse and I checked and prepared the drugs. The patient rushed in was a child, which intensified the situation. As the doctor started to ask for the drugs to be drawn up and ready to give, I turned to find SN had vanished. It was a nightmare scenario for me, I realised the drug vials attached directly to the syringe, instead of drawing up, and I didn't know how to do it. The doctor shot over and grabbed what he needed. SN never did return, so I felt completely useless. In school I had been assured that after every crash call the staff got together to debrief. The debrief seldom happened in practice, and I could have really done with it.

From casualty there arose the opportunity to spend time in x-ray, and the plaster room. In x-ray there would be a steady stream of patients that came to the department clutching their cards, and needed to be organised with a gown depending on the area to be xrayed. If the patient was elderly this could be an undertaking, as they often had layers of clothes to come off. The same applied in the plaster room, run by two men that had been there for years, had a great camaraderie with each other, and treated students with equal ease. The plaster of Paris, obedient in their hands, went everywhere with mine, and such good fun. To start with the saw to remove the plaster sounded and looked horrendous. Jim explained that the small circular saw did not spin, but oscillated very fast through the plaster, and would not cut the skin, something I soon got the hang of. Due to the dust from the plaster of Paris the pair had negotiated a milk ration as a perk of the job. One of them poked his head round the curtain while I attended a patient, and said he needed me for an oesophageal irrigation. Wondering what we going to do, he ushered me into the staff room for a cup of tea!. Shortly after my placement these two gentlemen disappeared under a bit of a cloud, I never did find out why.

Three years seemed a long time at the start of training, yet flew by, marked by gaining first my blue belt in the second year, and black belt in the third year, along with a smart RBH enamel badge for passing my hospital finals. (Both hospital finals and the enamel badge are no longer part of training). The first time I sat my states as they were called I failed, devastating at the time, I think I got the wrong end of the stick with a couple of the questions. Any way no problem second time round, much to my relief. I was offered a job on Hunter Ward by Sister D, who I got on well with, and so started my first post as a ward staff nurse on orthopaedic trauma.

Chapter 6: First Post

My nursing registration came through in the summer of 1981, and I could officially practice as a State Registered Nurse (now Registered General Nurse). I collected four new Staff Nurse dresses, saxe blue with white flashes on the collar from the sewing room. Once qualified we could wear a silver buckle attached to our black belt, earned in training. Mum gave me a lovely ornate ladies dress buckle that had been worn by my Grandmother in the early 1900s. Black tights and Lace up shoes completed the ensemble, and I started on Hunter Ward. Wages, paid monthly meant I started on about five to six hundred pounds a month. It doesn't sound much now, but to me it seemed a lot, prior to my training I had earned ten pounds a week as a mothers live in help. My first pay slip as a student was for seventy pounds, I bought a piece of cheesecake from the delicatessen on the King's Road to celebrate.

It seemed strange to move from the sheltered position of Student, to qualified nurse, and the feeling you should know everything, of course you don't, and every newly qualified nurse has this period of adjustment, mentored by a more experienced nurse. Under the watchful eye of Sister D my confidence built up, and I could run the ward for a shift, and knew I could refer to a senior if I needed to. The No7, Mrs K, or a sister acting up would tour the hospital each day, and check all ran smoothly, and collect statistics.

Mrs K, a tall angular lady with a shapeless suit was rather a nervous person. She said to the staff she tried to learn to drive, and her husband bought her a car that she was frightened of. She kept it at home, and gave it a little pat as she went past to catch the train to work each morning. Always made me smile.

The consultant's rounds happened three times a week. On Monday morning the senior consultant Mr C and his team came round before lunch. The medical entourage would be led by the senior nurse, who introduced each person to remind them of name age diagnosis. Progress would then be discussed, and I made a list of investigations and instructions to be carried out. One ward round we were making the transition from task orientated nursing, to patient centred nursing process. The role of the lead nurse on a shift changed to facilitator, and the patients divided between the trained staff on duty, so all needs for that patient were looked after by one nurse. Mr C started the round with my patients, and at the end of my two bays, I said:

"And now Mr C due to the nursing process I will hand you over to my colleague for the next group of patients". He responded as I thought he might:

"Nursing process, what the hell is that, where's sister?"

In the patient notes he wrote as he thought. Sister D suggested to him there was perhaps a more appropriate way of saying a patient was immobile, than writing: "This old girl is about as mobile as a jelly in summer". He paused and said yes there probably was, and his note writing modified after that. Like it or not he had to get used to the new way of working, and the many changes that came to the nurses he worked with. I heard years later that he had a terminal illness, Sister D went to see him in Dunedin, the local private hospital. He asked sister to look at his bottom, where he had a pressure ulcer (bed sore). Soon after he died, a sad end to a long and distinguished career. However he does now have a ward named after him at the RBH.

The other two orthopaedic consultants were debonair and self assured, as they moved swiftly from bed to bed with their registrar, and houseman. Mr A prided himself in the length of time he took to perform a total hip replacement, and in his spare time he played the saxophone at international level. Mr Co, tall and good looking with blond hair had a special interest in sports injuries, and ran a private clinic in this speciality. All the consultants did private work along side their NHS duties, and still do.

Each day the house officer would be round to clerk new patients, review the drug charts and make necessary addition or subtraction to the regime for each patient. These doctors, early in their training relied quite a bit on the trained staff on the ward at the beginning of their placement. It would be common for the trained nurse to suggest a certain medication and dose that would be used by his team. We would also keep a weather eye out for any discrepancy in a drug dose and point it out, the reason why it is so important for a trained nurse to be familiar with drug and dose that are used frequently. The drug charts were also checked every day by a trained pharmacist, so all staff worked together to make sure the patient received correct medication.

The drug round would be carried out by two trained nurses, then it was decided one nurse could do this on her own. Round we went with the drug trolley four times a day, breakfast, lunch, tea and bedtime. Before the start of a round I would try and make sure all the medications required were in the trolley, as it was time consuming if you had to go back to the stock cupboard. Every patient wore an identification band on their wrist, this along with asking their name went to ensure the right patient got the right drugs, and it would be signed off on the yellow drug sheet. After the round there would be the intravenous antibiotics, and once during the shift the controlled drugs needed to be checked for stock control.

Documentation is part and parcel of nursing, and is a working, legal record of everything that happens to each patient. To try and ensure all is clear and concise, it is a victim of its own making, in the effort for clarity and precision a nursing record has become increasingly complex. For years the Kardex system pervaded. A bit like a metal phone directory it had stepped leaves A-Z, and a card for each patient, with name, age, diagnosis, consultant, drugs and allergies. The ongoing record below had to be written at the end of each shift. Day shift was written in blue, and night shift in red, so easy to read. The problem with this record was it could be very repetitive, and might read something like this:

All care given, mobilised to toilet, fluids encouraged (blue ink)
Slept well (red ink).
Seen by Dr, no change, continues to mobilise (blue ink).
Slept well (red ink).
Eating well, mobility improved according to physio (blue ink).
Slept well, settled late (red ink).

These repetitive entries were not very meaningful, what did "all care" mean exactly? How many times did that patient go out to the toilet, once or ten times?. For this reason and in line with the nursing process the Kardex became the patient care-plan. Now each patient had an individualised careplan with shift notes, in an A4 folder at the end of the bed, instead of the Kardex kept at the nurses station. On admission a detailed history would be taken to ascertain what was normal for that person. This entailed a further new addition to nursing, a nursing model, a framework with which to plan care, and ensure no aspect got forgotten. There were various models, some suited to adult nursing, or psychiatry, children and so on.

At the RBH everyone used Elements of Nursing model (called The Elephants of Nursing by my son!), by Roper Tierney, and Logan. This model had twelve aspects of daily living, mobility, personal hygiene, breathing, eliminating, eating and so on. Each of these twelve areas then had physical, social, environmental, cultural and psychological factors applied, and underlying all, the birth to death continuum line, as the activities would be differently managed according to age. For example a physical aspect of eating for someone with no teeth, meant they would need a soft diet. If their hands had arthritis an environment to enable them to eat with special cutlery would be arranged to make sure they got enough food. With elimination on the continuum line, urinary output and kidney function would reduce naturally with age, to be expected as a normal part of the ageing progress.

All twelve activities of living were written in their appropriate boxes in the careplan, the idea being that one signature from the nurse looking after the patient would be made at the end of the shift, cutting down on the repetition of the Kardex, and on time. The complexity of the new records never quite achieved either, and nursing records have been constantly reviewed and changed ever since. Each page in the careplan had its own plastic document sleeve, this meant it had to be taken out, written on, and put back in, another little time trap in a busy day. The use of red ink for the night shift and blue for the day shift stopped as it was difficult to photocopy, and faded in old records, should they be needed in a court of law. All records now had to be in black ink. Litigation in nursing has escalated over the years, and a good set of nurse records will prove that a nurse has completed the duties she says she has, so are an absolute must, regardless of time.

While on the subject of records, the intravenous antibiotics were removed from the yellow drug chart, to a separate green chart with three sections. By this time I had passed my intravenous drug certificate, and the separation of the charts did help clarity. The medical records of each patient were in a buff folder, and bought up from medical records, and archived back there once the patient had been discharged. Some of these folders were huge, and occasionally two were needed, as the patient frequently came into hospital. I found some transparent plastic cards with small squares in the back of some notes. Sister explained they were a system called Microfisch and contained micronised notes. This initiative had been tried at some stage to reduce the storage required for notes. It seemed a good idea, but required a reader lamp to enlarge the text on the film. Every time the doctor wanted to see the notes, he had to go back to the lamp, so it didn't catch on, and no doubt cost a lot of money.

Chapter 7: Blood Everywhere

Elderly women with a fractured neck of femur (hip) were frequently admitted after a fall. Post menopause women are more prone to this type of fracture due to lack of oestrogen, hence the higher number of women than men that suffer this injury. The hip pain as the muscles contracted round the fracture was relieved once on the ward with temporary traction, prior to surgical repair. The hip would be repaired with a pin and plate, dynamic hip screw, Thompson or Austin Moore prosthesis, dependent on the position of the fracture. Temporary traction came as a kit, the adhesive bandage applied hip to ankle on the out side of the leg passed under the foot with a spacer, and the other end of the bandage stuck from ankle to groin on the inside of the leg. Then a spiral bandage from ankle to groin round the leg held all in place. The rope attached to the bottom of the foot spacer, hung over the end of the bed on a swan-neck pulley with a weight holder tied to the end. Each grey disk inserted weighed a pound, seven pounds would be the usual amount, or five pounds for a tiny lady. The effect of the weight would pull the ends of the bones back into line and reduce the pain

As soon as possible the patient went down to theatre, though there might be a wait of several days. Medical fitness for surgery frequently caused the delay, for example, their diabetes needed better control, or more acute emergencies occupied theatre time. In the case of a theatre emergency the delay, was not good for the patient, as the sooner they had surgery and got up the better, and frustrating for us. The patient, starved pre-med' given, and ready on a canvas to go to theatre, would be cancelled at the last minute. The pre-medication was always by injection, now the medication is given by mouth, as the small amount of water to swallow the tablets has been proved safe prior to anaesthesia.

The operation complete, recovery would ring the ward and request a nurse to collect the patient. The details of the operation, IV (intravenous) regime, and Redivac drain handed over, and back to the ward we went. The patient would be observed made comfortable, and the IV run according to the prescription. There were no pumps to regulate the rate, except in Intensive Care. So we all had a wooden tongue depressor with the different hourly drip rates written down kept to hand in our top pocket. The rate, regulated by a roller switch on the line, while timing the drops with a second hand, had to be watched in case the fluid ran through too fast or slow. If a patient, confused after anaesthetic pulled the cannulae out, it could be messy especially if a blood transfusion was running. The doctor would be called to replace the cannulae. Once I saw a SN mistake her clamp for her scissors, and instead of clamping the line, cut clean through it, blood everywhere. The Redivac, to drain blood from the operation site usually came out after twenty four hours, a bit longer if needed, again this could be subject to unscheduled removal due to confusion. A particularly confused lady we had succeeded in removing drip, drain, dressing and sutures, and had to go back to theatre to be re sutured.

Bandages used for traction, or to hold a dressing in place had to be hand washed and rolled ready for reuse. There were a lot, and hand washing wet, and time consuming, sister who hated waste insisted. I suggested to her that a small work top washing machine could be bought with ward funds, so we did, closely followed by a spin dryer. Washing was still a performance, though easier than by hand. I usually did it after lunch in a free side room, and hung the bandages on the radiator to dry. Eventually infection control stepped in and decreed the bandages must be thrown away after single use. I don't know what happened to our machine or spin dryer, probably gathering dust somewhere

The other type of traction commonly used was a Thomas splint for fractured shaft of femur (thigh bone), the principal of pain relief being the same as for a neck of femur. This splint , invented in the First World War remained unchanged in design and purpose. It consisted of a metal leather covered ring that should fit snugly but not to tight round the groin and top of the thigh. From the ring, a metal loop followed the leg from the groin, round the foot, and re-joined the ring on the hip side of the leg. The loop, prepared with short lengths of pale green wool baise bandage, would be pinned with safety pins from side to side, and then gamgee tissue laid on top to support the leg. Two of us then gently slid the prepared splint up the leg to the groin , this allowed the leg to rest on the sling created by the baise and gamgee. A metal Steinman or Denham pin inserted in theatre through the tibia below the knee or calcaneus (heel bone), took traction weights of up to twelve pounds on ropes over the end of the bed. The foot of the bed was raised to give counter traction, and stop the patient being pulled down the bed by the traction weights. Supported from the overhead bed rails by further ropes attached to a three way pulley and counter weight, the splint gave the patient movement in bed. It allowed them movement up the bed to get on to a bedpan, and nurses to change the bottom sheet etc, without disturbing the fracture. Bone healing took twelve weeks.

People that came in with a fractured femur tended to be young, the injury sustained from a sports injury, such as a fall from a horse, contact sports, or a road traffic accident. At one time we had two young girls opposite each other on their twelve weeks of traction. One a traffic accident, and the other more unusual. From a well off Asian family Hermione, at private school had increasing thigh pain, and was sent to the doctor, who requested an x-ray. A sarcoma, a bone cancer diagnosed, she had extensive surgery to remove the cancer. Her elderly and naturally worried parents flew in from Asia, and had anxious words with the consultant. In fact both these teenagers did very well, settled in to their enforced bed rest, played their music, became friends and varnished their nails. As an anaesthetists said as one of then lay in recovery, one of the worlds beautiful people, and this true of both girls. They got better and carried on their lives.

When the time came for the traction to be taken down, and the pin removed after twelve weeks, we usually did this in the morning. The patient would be given a small amount of oral sedation, and the pin pulled out on the ward, with a T-handle attached to the end of the pin. A firm pull and twist, in the case of a Denham pin removed it with minimum discomfort, and the small puncture wounds healed in a few days. Occasionally pin removal did not go to plan. One lady had a below knee plaster on, with a pin through the plaster and heel. When I tried to pull it out on the count of three as normal, no amount of pulling and twisting had any effect. In theatre later, the surgeon found that the cotton wool lining of the plaster had twisted round the pin, and stopped removal. Now free of traction the physio would have the patients standing, walking, and home in a few days.

One young man that sticks in my mind had come in with a femoral fracture, and developed a suspected DVT, (deep vein thrombosis, a clot), in his leg. To confirm this, I took him for a scan of the leg, in the scan department in North Wing, the old part of the hospital. An undertaking on a hospital bed, as the doctor did not want the traction disturbed if possible, so the strings were tied off to the end of the Thomas splint, otherwise the weights would swing and bang on the bed. Dave and I duly set off with two porters wheeling the bed. Dave had a red blanket over him as there was some distance to the scan room. We descended in the lift to ground floor of South Wing, then out through plastic doors into the link corridor.

The link corridor ran from one end of the hospital site to the other and joined all departments. It had a corrugated flat roof, and opaque plastic sides mounted on a metal frame, the floor was either painted cement or paving slabs, and no insulation or heating. We trundled along past the exits to the kitchen and maternity block on the right, through eye block that also housed main x-ray. On to Nuffield block, with three gynae wards and Kempton, the children' Ward on the right. (Named after Dr Kempton, I attended a clinic appointment in the 1960s with my mother, Dr Kempton failed to turn up, and tragically had drowned at sea with all hands). Then down hill, and up hill past Victoria on the left, and Benyon the other side, and a sharp turn to the left brought us into the main hall of the old hospital. The scan facility, in a room on the right just past the double oak front door came into view. A huge problem arose, try as we might, the bed proved too long for the corridor to turn into the doorway, that was too narrow.

After much scratching of heads it proved impossible, no-one had presented in a bed before, patients always came on a trolley, so back to the ward we went. The scan had to be done, so after all, the traction was taken down, with the pin tied off to the bottom of his Thomas splint, and Dave carefully manoeuvred on to a stretcher and slid onto a trolley. The scan proved positive, and he started his anticoagulant therapy for his DVT. After twelve weeks he went home, and we heard later that he had had a pulmonary embolus (clot in his lung), and died. An awful outcome after all the effort he and the staff had put into his recovery.

Chapter 8: Optional Extras and Emergency Take

With a variety of other types of trauma injury admitted, a patient might have what we flippantly called "optional extras", diabetes, stroke, Parkinson's and so on. Hazel came in with a fractured hip, and suffered a stroke during her surgery. She was quite switched off, so rehab took a long time. Her left side proved no use to her at all, making all activities of daily living very difficult. To begin with her swallowing put her at risk of aspiration pneumonia, where food goes into the lungs, so nasogastric feeding helped to prevent this. There were no balanced feeds then, or the feeding pumps for increased accuracy and control.

The nasogastric tube, thicker than the modern micro bore ones, had the end spigoted off between meals, and the tube hung behind an ear. Each meal time the spigot was replaced with a large syringe, so Buildup, Complan or liquefied food poured into the syringe funnel, went into the stomach by gravity. Before doing this a small amount of gastric contents were aspirated, and tested with litmus paper for acidity, to check the tip of the nasogastric tube rested in the stomach. After each feed ten mils of water would be flushed through to clean the tube. When the nasogastric tube came out and Hazel ate, food packed in her cheeks like a squirrel, and her weight increased alarmingly as she seemed to be in eating auto pilot mode. The left hand side of Hazel's body, completely dense with no feeling was a dreadful handicap. Despite conscientious use of Bobath positions, especially designed to improve limb awareness, the method did little to help in this respect, and is no longer used.

It became obvious Hazel would not be able to look after herself, and off she went to a nursing home. You never know with a stroke how a person will do. In my training on Castle at Battle, a lady came in unconscious and we thought she might die. By morning she had woken up, and apart from a slight slur in her speech went home fully mobile a week later

One young man admitted via casualty came to the ward with an unusual injury. He had been out cycling on a racing bike, had come off, and the break lever had ended up embedded in his thigh. In this type of injury the foreign body needs to be removed with great care under general anaesthetic, because it may have penetrated a blood vessel or nerve path. If pulled out a major bleed or severe damage to other structures could occur. At the scene of the accident the rest of the bike had been cut away by the fire brigade, and the ambulance crew had stabilised the break lever in the thigh, for the trip to casualty. When he arrived on the ward, and the dressing carefully removed for pre theatre inspection for the registrar, it looked really weird sticking at right angles from the thigh. Luckily no major injury had occurred when the lever was removed, and he soon went home to recover while the wound healed.

Alice was admitted on emergency take, (taken in turn with Lister and Heygroves Ward), with a fractured neck of femur. I started to admit her in side room one behind the nurses station, as the only bed available. Alice was elderly, polite and chatty, and played down the seriousness of her injury. We went through her personal details, history, and completed her property list. I asked a colleague to come and help me undress her, as I could see this would be difficult on my own. Alice became increasingly agitated as I explained we would need to get her into a nightie so the doctor could fully examine her. We gently insisted and the layers of clothing were stripped away. Elderly people specialise in many layers of clothing, cardigan, dress, petticoat, vest, bra and knickers all had to be removed, difficult with someone with reduced mobility flat in her bed. We got to the tight pink petticoat, and the material appeared stained over the left breast. Very embarrassed Alice made light of it.

Our suspicions were confirmed by an increasing odour as her bra came off. This revealed a horrendous fungating breast wound, an extensive area of broken skin with deep slough and necrotic (dead) tissue. She had tried to manage the wound herself and had not wanted to bother the doctor. It was no surprise when the cause of her hip fracture turned out to be pathological, a secondary cancer of the bone. The wound was dressed, and Alice started on regular Mixt Bromptoms, a morphine and alcohol mix used at the time for cancer pain. Alice quickly deteriorated, and said to sister: "Am I going to die?". In her candid way sister sat with her, and commented that everyone would die one day, and to make the most of each day as it came. Over the next few days Alice seemed more accepting and calmer before she died.

When a patient died on the ward, the side room door would be shut, or the curtains drawn round the other beds in the bay if the person died there. They would be laid flat, arms straight either side, eyelids closed, and a pillow under the chin if the jaw had a tendency to drop. Once the doctor had certified the death the patient could be prepared for the mortuary. Two of us stocked the back trolley, with the addition of the laying out equipment kept in a Huntley's biscuit tin. The person, washed head to toe, had a swab of cotton wool placed in the rectum, and any other orifice that required one. This was done with a pair of red plastic forceps. A long sleeved paper gown with ruffles sewn down the front would then be put on. If there were dentures they were inserted in the mouth to keep facial shape, and hair combed. In the early days of my career the jaw was bandaged shut with a crepe bandage over the top of the head, the bandage left facial marks, hence a pillow below the jaw in place of the bandage. The great toes, tied together, had a brown card label attached with name, date of birth, time and date of death. Then a clean bed sheet placed under the body would be folded down over the face, and up over the feet, and the sides drawn over the torso, right to left and left to right. Around the shoulders, hips and ankles a cotton bandage secured the shroud, with a further label taped to the chest with the same details as the one on the toes. A third clean sheet would then be placed over the body and the bed. An air of calm enveloped the room once it had been tidied, and a small posy of flowers placed on the locker next to the bed. The porters came up with the mortuary trolley, thinly disguised under a red blanket, to collect the body. Details handed over, included presence of a pace maker, as the mortuary staff have to remove the device to stop it exploding in cremation.

Death on a ward is a sad time primarily for the relatives, who may be with the patient as they died, or wish to see the body before it goes to the mortuary. It is also sad for the surrounding patients as despite the curtains it was obvious that someone had died. The staff felt sad for the patient, relatives and surviving patients, and often a sense of relief knowing that the person died peacefully, and no longer suffered.

Other taxing events involved patients who for what ever reason became disruptive and difficult to manage round the other patients and ward routine. Boulder, a man from Czechoslovakia, who lived at Burrough Court came on to the ward. Somehow he had jumped out of the first floor lavatory window, and fractured both calcaneus (heel bones) as he landed.

He had severe learning difficulties, and careful management by the learning disability team gave the only way his violent and unpredictable behaviour could be controlled. Of all the injuries he might have sustained, as far as we were concerned he had the ideal one for a general hospital. The pain in both heels meant he was completely bed bound and unable to stand, far less walk about. He shouted a great deal, and thankfully had a nursing member from Borough Court with him all the time, until he went back there.

There were humorous moments. One day a well known comedian visited the hospital on a cheering up mission. When he got to Hunter the staff had been warned of his arrival, and we greeted him with the biggest syringe available, and pretended to mistake him for a patient. The patients were in on the prank, and I think he found it funny as well. One of the tasks of cleaning at the weekend was to collect all glass thermometers in their plastic holders to be washed, dried and returned to the wall by each bed. A wonderful story circulated that a student nurse then did a denture round, and gathered every ones dentures in a bowl, together as she had the thermometers. Imagine the chaos it caused.

Another incident occurred with a lady in the side room behind the nurses station, these rooms were used if the patient had an infection, or poorly. A couple of times we heard a low buzzing noise from the room, and thought nothing of it. However when sister went in for something she found a vibrator in the fruit bowl. Of course we found this terribly funny, and all had to go into the room on a pretence to have a look, and sure enough there it was!

In one of the six bedded bays there was a little old lady who had been in for weeks, she would roll up small bits of her faeces in paper, and put them in the locker. When staff tried to talk to her about this, she denied all knowledge and blamed the dog. The other live wire was Jim call me Lillian. He would walk through from Lister Ward next door, and proclaim to anyone around: "I have the body of a man, but the mind of a women, call me Lillian". He lived out in the sticks and had taken to riding his bicycle along the main road, dressed in a frock, high heels and a long wig, waving and jeering at any cars that tooted. At home he lived alone and lived entirely on baked beans heated in a microwave. The inevitable happened and he got knocked off his cycle, hence his admission.

In 1983 I became pregnant, and decided that once my baby was born, I would carry on working full time on day duty. It took a bit of organisation, and eventually Alistair and I lined up a child minder we both liked, that didn't smoke, and was not wrapped up in their own baby. I continued to work up to six weeks before my due date, and planned to return to work five weeks after the birth, normal maternity leave at that time. I have always been fit, and carried on riding at home, and working without any problem until my maternity leave started. You could have maternity dresses, but I found I didn't need one.

Charles Merlin -Charlie was born at the end of November, and as planned I started back at work. Our routine at home ran something like this. On an early shift I would get Charlie washed dressed and fed, express milk for later, and Alistair dropped him at the child minder, I collected him on my way home at about four. On a late shift I dropped him on the way in at lunchtime, and Alistair would pick him up at about five. I had planned to continue riding my Honda 90, but the logistics became too complicated as I needed to drop Charlie off by car and return home for the bike, so I sold it. End of an era, as I had had two Honda 50s, a 70 then the 90 since I left school. Reliable and cheap to run, at fifty pence a week, I rode my bike in all weathers. I did come off on the ice a couple of times, apart from a black elbow, which sister said I was lucky not to have broken, I avoided any serious injury. Alistair could see the headlight of the bike coming over the bridge after a late shift, and knew to get supper on the table.

Chapter 9: All Change

The first time I became directly affected by government intervention came when all staff that worked for the NHS had to be re-graded. Instead of a one two three system, A to H would be used. In my naivety and everyone else's, we all assumed a simple swap from number to letter. Not so, as of course the exercise was to slightly down grade as many people as possible and save on the wages bill. So instead of the expected E grade, I and many others received D grade in our letter. Then it was down to us to prove we were worth the E grade. It caused a huge amount of upset and disillusionment, and hard work. I had to trawl through dozens of old Kardex, to find the dates I had, for example been next door to Gauvain Ward, to give paediatric IV antibiotics. Some of these records had mysteriously disappeared. As a trained nurse I had joined the Royal College of Nursing (RCN) for indemnity insurance. This meant an RCN representative attended my hearing with me, and my D was upgraded to an E, as the panel agreed I worked at the required level.

Up until the time of re-grading there had always been a senior and a junior sister on each ward. With the cost saving exercise of grading, each ward from now on would have one sister. Sister D, dug her toes in, so Sister B who had been there longer had to move into the vacancy on Lister. No one liked the idea of only one sister per ward, but there was no choice in the matter.

Other changes that came in the mid 1980s began to come thick and fast. The care of pressure areas (bed sores), were first in line. Little had changed in the management of these debilitating injuries since Florence Nightingale identified them as a problem, and were frequently seen as inevitable in someone that had taken to their bed. New research showed that practices believed to be good, created problems. The first to go was the draw sheet and plastic underneath, tucked across to protect the bottom sheet, and allow an easy change if the patient was incontinent. The thick cotton of the draw sheet could graze the skin, and the plastic underneath had the potential to cause sweating and skin maceration. The draw sheets were also used to haul people up the bed, not an intended use, all were banished, and incontinence managed with modern nappy pads. For the same risk to skin, the old disposable grey paper and plastic incontinence sheets could no longer be used under a person.

New research revealed that sheepskin seat and heel pads should be used as comfort aids only as they did not in fact relieve pressure. Another common practice had been to fill a rubber glove with water tied off to form a little cushion. This would then be placed one under each heel, it was proved ineffective for pressure relief, and had no business in modern care. Both were replaced with static low air appliances such as Roho cushions and heel boots. The red rubber inflatable doughnut cushion went, as it concentrated skin pressure where the buttocks dropped through the hole, replaced by thick foam cushions with a waterproof cover, and a pillow case over the top. There were a number of innovative beds, the Flotron, very heavy as it was filled with sand, that circulated under a membrane, by electric pump, and in effect kept the patient airborne. The net bed that attached to a normal bed had a frame with a net suspended from it, and a handle at each corner, so the patient could be easily turned from side to side. It proved difficult to use, and left net marks on the skin, this bit of kit soon disappeared.

Then the first generation of the modern pressure relief mattresses used today began to come on the scene, it gave a big improvement on the old ripple mattress that was the only one available. I remember having a stand up row with a particularly bossy sister that was covering, who still insisted on two hourly turns at night. I pointed out to her that the whole ethos behind the mattress, was that it relieved pressure by constantly alternating air pressure, and this protected the skin and allowed the person to have a proper nights sleep. We had a good ding dong over a patient, very unprofessional, but I just saw red.

Standard Invacare and Hoskins Kings Fund beds were not replaced by the modern hospital beds, controlled with an electric handset, until well after I left the hospital. Everything on the Hoskins / Invacare beds was manually operated. The backrest had an awkward catch to release, and with a heavy patient, pillows and all proved a real wrestling match to adjust. The foot of the bed had a lever to elevate it, and the bed raised and lowered with a hydraulic foot pump underneath. On each wheel a break could be applied, stiff and difficult to operate when the wheel stuck in a certain position.

Along side the new equipment came the start of a revolution in wound care dressings. The last true innovation had been the invention of paraffin gauze, Jelonet in the First World War, the first attempt to try and prevent the dressing sticking to the wound. Before this, clean lint or gauze used on the wound, dried and stuck, making removal very painful, and disrupted healing. Gauze strips soaked in EUSOL (Exeter University Solution of Lime) or EUSOL and paraffin, had been the only packing available for years, for deep wounds to stop them healing superficially with a cavity underneath.

The first new dressing we had on Hunter was Granuflex, a hydrocolloid that not only did not stick to the wound, but also created an ideal healing environment with optimum temperature, humidity and pain relief at dressing changes. It took a bit of getting used to, as when it came off a funny smell, and brown goo had to be cleaned away, we soon realised that wounds responded quickly, and pain reduced. A two part foam solution came onto the market in place of gauze packing, that had to be mixed together and poured into the wound cavity, and removed to be washed and replaced. Our test one made in its little round pot, looked like a willy, displayed proudly on the nurses station. Seaweed packing Kaltostat, soon followed, completely biodegradable it caused no wound trauma on removal, the surgeons took a bit of persuasion to stop using gauze, but eventually saw the benefits. Dressing removal ready for the doctor's round stopped, as the wound was unnecessarily exposed, and took several hours to return to optimum healing temperature when recovered with a fresh dressing.

The dressing packs that came up form CSSD were discontinued. They contained a round plastic galley pot, five cotton wool balls, five gauze swabs a surgipad, and plastic rubbish bag. A pack, placed on the bottom shelf of a metal dressing trolley cleaned with chlorhexidine, would be bought to the patients bedside. After hand washing the pack was opened on the top shelf of the trolley. The old dressing was removed with the red pair of forceps, and wound cleaned with cotton wool balls soaked in saline from the galley pot, held by the green forceps. A seperate wet ball was used either side and down the middle of the wound, then a dry one either side. Forceps fiddly to use went out when the CSSD packs were discontinued. Instead gloved hands to hold the gauze for cleaning, proved easier and offered less risk of trauma to the wound bed. Gauze replaced cotton wool, as gauze reduced   fibre deposits in the wound, and dressing packs became disposable

If a patient had diabetes their urine would be regularly tested to see if their blood glucose remained in normal range, and no ketones were present. Abnormality of either can cause coma in its most severe form, and will delay healing and the patient would be at higher risk of stroke, renal failure or heat attack. The test kit kept in a small wooden cupboard in the sluice, contained glass test tubes, and two tubes of tablets, one to test for glucose, the other for ketones. A pipette full of urine added to two test tubes would then have a glucose tablet added to one, and a ketone tablet to the other. The colour change then indicated the range, blue for normal, and stages of orange if glucose was present, and ketone level, indicated by increasing mauve colour. Estimation of blood glucose is more accurate if a blood sample is used, as glucose that is excreted in the urine is an old measure of what the level of glucose was

When we first had the test strips to do this, the only glucometer available in South Wing resided in ICU (Intensive Care Unit). A sample of blood, would be taken by pricking the finger with a sterile needle, (special finger pricking devices had not yet been invented). Then test strip in hand we had to run round to ICU to use the glucometer, or the sample became too old. The machine, awkward to use often showed error, this meant starting all over again. Laughable when I think of it now, but that is how it was. Today there are a plethora of modern machines, easy to use and much more accurate.

Health and safety became increasingly formalised. If a glass thermometer or syphgmonometer broke the mercury would escape and roll round the floor. A special kit for mercury spillage was introduced, it contained an apron, gloves, a paper cup to catch the mercury with, and a special box for disposal. At school in chemistry most pupils of my era had the chance to obtain a small piece of mercury, and pour it from hand to hand, or chase it round the desk with a pencil, oblivious to any risk.

Among the staff on Hunter there was a happy camaraderie, most of us worked full time, with a few part-timers, and with a separate staff for night duty there was no internal rotation. Our senior staff nurse ran the ward with a calm hand, and seemed ready for a sister's post. Then there were the four of us more junior SNs. We all had our little niches. K, really good at the off duty, spent a great deal of time over it, regardless of other things that went on. Doing the off duty never appealed to me, and I avoided it most of my time in nursing. It could take hours to safely fill the shifts, taking into account holiday, requests for particular days off and so on. Then altered due to last minute events, such as sickness, transport difficulties, childcare etc. Thankfully none of us were often sick, and would come in if at all possible. C came to the team after me, she had worked in Saudi Arabia and had all sorts of interesting anecdotes. Their shifts were divided into three lots of eight hours in twenty four, which avoided the long tiring night shifts of UK hospitals, very sensible. S lived in one of the outlying villages, and had several dogs that always caused her one problem or another.

State Enrolled nurses of the team included two full timers, one converted to State Registered, and eventually moved, and two who worked part time and worked two days a week, and C four days. B had an ailing husband who must have been very hard work, I had a soft spot for her, as she was so anxious and worried about everyone's wellbeing despite her own difficulties.

Time went on, and my second baby was born. I worked up to six weeks before the birth, as with Charlie. On maternity leave I carried on doing the usual things at home. The day Georgette was born, I attended clinic in the morning, and said to the Doctor I had had twinges overnight. She examined me and reported nothing much was happening yet, I remember thinking: "It is my second baby, but you're the Doctor". Dad came over for lunch, and afterwards I took him and Charlie out driving with Star my pony. The contractions got stronger, making me hang on to the reins and driving whip until they passed. Dad went home, and as Alistair came in from work, I told him we had to leave for the maternity unit right now. Off we went, he driving through the traffic, while advising me to pant or puff or what ever I was meant to do. On arrival he calmly walked into reception and said he needed the team who delivered babies in the car. Everyone came rushing out, helped me out of the car, and said to keep my legs together as we went up in the lift. Georgette was born ten minutes later after a couple of breaths of Entonox. Like Charlie another lovely healthy baby. All the girls came over from Hunter to see her, as they did when Charlie came along.

This time I decided to come back part time on night duty. To pay for two lots of childcare was not worth while, and I wanted to be home more with the children. With the enhanced hours of night duty, I could earn almost the same as full time day duty doing two nights a week. These were split nights as I did not feel I could do two in a row with both little ones. My ward became Lister next door to Hunter, as the part time vacancy was there.

Chapter 10: Night Duty

I returned to work as planned, and caused a bit of a stir. Georgette, like Charlie had started sleeping through the night by six weeks, so tongue in cheek I suggested to night sister that I bring her in to sleep in a side room, so I could carry on breast feeding. Sister nearly had a fit at such an idea, my request had been taken at face value. Plan B sprang into action, I left expressed breast milk for Alistair to settle her and give breakfast. The first night was a real endurance test for me, I steeled myself to be alert and functioning when all I wanted to do was go to bed. I took each hour one at a time, and had a sleep on my break at two in the morning. After revival with Horlicks and toast the night went on, dawn came and then early morning duties, drug round, handover, and home!

The night shift started with report from the day shift, then out on the ward to settle people down for the night, we aimed to get the main lights out by about ten thirty, eleven o'clock. The day staff had given hot drinks at about eight pm, this consisted of a trolley with all manor of powdered drinks, a large kettle of hot water, and hot milk heated in the ward kitchen with a double saucepan, to prevent burning the milk on the bottom of the pan. Each patient would be offered a hot drink of their choice, coffee, tea, chocolate Horlicks. Overtime, Bovril, Marmite, cold or hot milk. Horlicks and Oveltine required a special cylindrical blue plastic jug with posher, supplied by Horlicks to make the perfect malty milk drink. Powdered drink added to hot milk in the jug received a vigorous beating up and down with the posher to produce a foaming and delicious hot drink, great fun to make. The only really disgusting drink as far as I was concerned, was if a patient asked for hot Bovril made with milk, I couldn't imagine anything worse. At one stage it was decreed that ward kitchen stock would be discontinued, and a Maxpax vending machine trialled. Patients would be able to get a hot drink when they felt like one, any time of day or night. Drinks were watery and insipid compared with those on a drinks trolley, and many of the patients could not access the machine due to bed rest or poor mobility. The drinks trolley was reinstated.

Normally there would be two or three of us on duty, two trained and a night auxiliary, or sometimes two of us, one trained. At hand over we decided who would do what, and start work. It varied on how busy the ward turned out on a shift due to a variety of circumstance. A full ward, take nights, two or more patients who needed hourly or more frequent attention, meant a busy night with little respite. On the other hand the night could pass peaceably enough, and be rather boring, though reading and quiet chatter helped a bit. Every hour each patient was checked, sometimes it would really seem as though a patient had stopped breathing, they were sleeping deeply really, and it always came as a relief when they finally took a breath. We would work our breaks out between us, and if possible take a bit longer if we could, several of us had young children, and it helped.

The problem with sleeping on a break, came if something happened and it was necessary to spring straight back into action, with no time to wake up properly. On one occasion a more junior member of staff woke me early from my break, as a patient had deteriorated after their hip operation earlier that day. The doctor on call had already arrived, and the patient needed complex observation, and urgent IV fluids set up as they were bleeding from the wound. Trying to get everything sorted out to stabilise the patient was not easy, while frantically gathering my wits from sleep mode.

Nights could be a long ordeal for patients too. A young man given a diagnosis of an aggressive osteosarcoma in his thigh had an agonising decision to make. His body scan proved negative, no cancer spread found in any other organ. A hind quarter amputation, major surgery where his leg would be amputated through the hip joint, was the only recommendation the surgical and oncology teams, after much discussion could offer. The poor chap had a dreadful sleepless night; all three of us on duty took it in turns to see if he wanted moral support between his fitful dozing. He made the brave choice to go ahead with the surgery. After a few nights in Intensive Care, he came back to Lister ward, very uncomfortable, and unable to get his balance. Unfortunately the post operative body scan showed extensive cancer spread in other organs, and he gave up the struggle, became palliative dying a couple of weeks later. Everyone felt very sad.

The ward lights would be put on at six in the morning, for early observations and drug round. At about five in the morning, to help the day staff, we had to wash and get up the four patients who needed most help. This meant a bed bath, then up in their chairs ready for breakfast, which was not until eight o'clock. People seldom get up this early, and to wake an elderly sometimes confused person at five was ridiculous. In line with the nursing process this practice stopped. Lights now came on at seven, and no one received an unnecessarily early wash, and the drug round became day routine. This is a good example of changes for the patients being made for the better, the day staff had to accommodate these duties as they had the staff on the morning shift. For those of us on night duty it was a great relief, and we could concentrate on patients that did need attention, and the other patients remained undisturbed.

As I worked part time, I often got moved to help out on Hunter, Trueter, Heygroves or the children's orthopaedic ward Gauvain, or Brodie ward. I did not mind, as I knew the other night staff, and it made a change. On Hunter, P coming up for retirement proved a real character. At midnight she liked to go on her break, as she relied on a good nip of sherry to get her through the night. If a patient crashed (collapsed), P had a real thing about resuscitation and calling the crash team out, she said nature should take its course, and one should turn a blind eye. For the rest of us knowing this it made an interesting shift, we would double check who had "Not for 2--" (the code used for resuscitation status), written in the notes, and kept a careful eye on those that were for resuscitation. At that time the medical team would make this decision, with seldom any reference to the patient or relatives concerned. Many years later in an effort to address this and include the patient, things have got terribly complicated and not much better.

While on Hunter, late one night I stood in the sluice that overlooked the service yard, and the vehicle entrance to the mortuary. A steady stream of black vans delivered multiple bodies into the building. It was unusual for there to be much action, but this particular night was after the gunman Michael Ryan went mad in Savernake Forest and Hungerford. He shot and killed sixteen people before police bought him down, or he shot himself, the truth of which is unknown. Sadly Sister Sue Godfrey, who I knew had lost her life, the mother of a young family, I had worked with her at Battle Hospital, everyone was shocked at what had happened. Alistair had heard the gunshots as he snoozed in the works van on Hungerford Warf, we had been very lucky. Near the end of my time on nights on Huntley and Palmer I had the police ring me. They were trying to gather any information about a dreadful incident that had happened at Burghfield Lock, a short distance from our house. Three young children from the same family had drowned in the lock, they had been under the care of their mother who had mental health problems. We had been out for the day, and had not seen them, and could not add to the investigation. Both the Hungerford shooting and the lock deaths bought a sinister and surreal feeling to those particular nights.

Gauvain and Brodie ward I went to less frequently. What stands out in my mind about Gauvain is the treatment room. Day sister, proactive in raising funds for her ward, achieved a large donation. This could have been from British Airways or a private sheik. The room had smart storage units, examination couch, and distraction mobiles, a masterpiece in design and must have cost a fortune. Eventually Gauvain closed, and amalgamated with Kempton. I wonder what became of that treatment room, I doubt if the sponsor knew what happened.

Brodie Ward, downstairs and next to casualty, took patients for over night observation, and day cases for minor surgery. One night that I helped out there, a man came in with confusion. He was on the go most of the night, and other than shepherd him about there was no way of keeping him in bed. He took off out of the ward with me in tow, and barged straight through casualty x-ray. The radiologist got very cross, I explained the difficulties we were having. Help from the porters had little effect, though we eventually got him back to the ward. We gave him a cup of tea, which he promptly took under the nurse's station, and stayed there for the remainder of the night wrapped in a red blanket.

On the whole I felt I coped well working nights, though tiredness sometimes got the better of me. When the children were both at home I tried to doze, while keeping an eye on them. I must have gone to sleep, and woke to find the front door open, Dashing out Charlie came up the path leading his little sister, and announced they had been for a walk round the island. Luckily as we lived on the river, they did not have the fascination for it that other children had. One day when they were both at school, and I dropped into bed dead tired, I woke, and saw that it was five o'clock, when I should have collected them at three thirty. I launched out of bed, got dressed, glanced at the clock, and saw I had mis-read five for eleven twenty five. Clothes off and straight back to sleep. The same morning I had clipped the wing mirror of a parked car on my way home driving from work, fortunately no damage done.

The temptation if something was going on after a night duty always caught me out. Both racing at Lockhinge, and a day out boating with friends became an endurance test for me. I tried to have quick naps so not to miss out and found firstly they made no difference at all, and secondly I was either too hot or too cold, my body thermostat unable to cope with fatigue. When Georgette was sixteen weeks old, and Charlie two years, we flew out to Alderney in the Channel Isles on holiday, after working the previous night. I fell asleep on the beach and sun burnt the backs of both my legs. Apart from that it was a super holiday and I walked everywhere with Georgette in a backpack.

I started to look at what else I could do, and decided to investigate community nursing. The years diploma course would give me a sister's post on a G grade, and the hours would fit in with family life reasonably well. Over the years since I qualified, I had completed three ENB (English National Board) modules, the post registration courses then. ENB 941 Care of the Elderly ENB 978 Continence Care, and ENB 931 Care of the Dying. After spending a day out with a district nurse, I applied for the course. The interview went well, though I did not get a place, as more recent study, and different ward experience was required.

I asked for a transfer to a medical ward, and moved to Huntley and Palmer in the old part of the hospital. The entrance to the ward, immediately off the main hall, displayed impressive nineteenth century architecture. From outside the hospital main entrance dominated the King's Road, the carved stone columns and stair case in bath stone, show cased the front door. In Elm house, where night sister's office was, there used to be a wonderful picture of a smart Hackney, put to a stick back gig, driven by a gentleman in a top hat, going past the front of the hospital. I hope this ended up in the hospital museum or library when Elm house was demolished. Through the main door the grand staircase swept up either side to wards, with the hospital chapel opposite the front door. In the stairwell hung a full size oil portrait of Lord Benyon and another benefactor that remain there to this day. Running along the entire length of the building in the basement, there is a corridor, and rooms off this contained the original hospital laundry, eerie at night, and the doors either end are now locked making this cut through much safer.

Huntley and Palmer mirrored the nightingale ward, Adelaide above, with the addition of a balcony, and had fewer beds. The access up four steps to the balcony meant it was impossible to get either the drugs trolley, or the crash trolley to the bedside. The least poorly slept here, in original old iron framed hospital beds, the type seen in comic strips, or charity bed pushes. Balcony beds, five in all, were cramped, cold in winter, hot in summer, yet the light flooded in through the single glazed windows, and promoted a microclimate of camaraderie between occupants. The staff had thoughtfully put a grow bag of tomatoes for the patients to tend. Huntley and Palmer took medical patients, including those needing dialysis, they would be on a Gambol, a complex temperamental machine that had a plethora of warning lights and buzzers. There were few at night who knew how to deal with it. The Gambol is no longer used, superseded by continuing ambulatory peritoneal dialysis that the patients do themselves at home.

At evening class at Reading College I completed a Sociology GCSE, and the City and Guilds Foundation Teaching and Assessment, with good grades. Sometimes I went straight to work from my class. A year later after re-application I obtained both a place and funding to start a Diploma in Community Nursing the following September, really good news. This period turned out to be one of a big high, followed by a big low for me. We had spent a great family Christmas together with Dad. Just after New Year in 1991 he was admitted to the Radcliffe in Oxford. Alistair and I visited him in CCU (coronary care unit), and he reported he had been very confused. He moved on to a medical ward to recover. One morning Myles my brother rang to say Dad had collapsed and died. A dreadful shock for us all.

After funeral arrangements and coming to terms with what happened, the year slid on by. At the end of August I worked my final night on Huntley and Palmer. As the pale light of dawn stole into the ward, I felt a mantle falling off my shoulders, and a huge feeling of relief. I vowed to myself that I would never stay up all night ever again. This I have remained true to, apart from one night last year when I found myself on Scarfell Pike at three thirty in the morning that is another story.

Chapter 11: Student District Nurse in Training

On the induction day for my new course I arrived at Bulmershe, the community faculty of Reading University in Woodley. The building, opened in the 1970s included a library, and printing/ arts department on site, this became very handy. This busy day contained meeting the rest of the nurses on the course, and receiving a mound of forms to deal with. The following day we were all teamed up with our CPT (clinical practice teacher), who would mentor for the practical elements of the course, sign off supervised practice, and be that all important person to turn to for reassurance and discussion. CPTs are district nursing isters (DNS) who have achieved a teaching qualification and can mentor DN students. My CPT was very skilled at this, and we remain friends to this day. Practical placements amounted to six weeks with your CPT before Christmas, and three months supervised practice at a different surgery, prior to qualifying. The rest of the year consisted of time in university, private study, and final exams of multiple choice and a written paper.

Study had become more academic since I completed nurse training, with written work needing to be properly referenced. This was all new to me, plus the fact computers were being used to search for information, instead of manually as I had been used to. The group had several library sessions about this, and how to use Word to write the work up. I had bought myself an electronic word processor so I didn't have to come into the library to work. Library computers were too few, and temperamental. The librarian did the searches, for the student to go through the list and decide which articles they wanted, and these were printed out. The four pieces of work included one on a nursing procedure, psychology, sociology and a final case study about a patient nursed during the course. My first, on different types of catheters had a mediocre mark, being descriptive in content. I soon learnt that academic work should be about comparison, contrast and conclusive discussion. No problem for the next three, and I passed with good grades.

My first week out on practical placement at Grovelands Surgery came. I had been looking forward to this, and as suspected nursing people at home is very different to a hospital environment. For a start patients were dressed, and in charge, we being a guest in their home. There was no clinical room or dressing trolley, and hand washing facilities varied, no ready supply of soap and hand towels, though most patients would supply a hand towel specifically for the nurse if requested. Nursing supplies had to be taken in to the house, and ordered via the surgery as needed. In place of the hospital stock cupboard, we all had a black leather district nursing bag. The bag was stocked with all kinds of dressings, bandages, catheters and so on, to avoid going back to the surgery, and enable us to deal with wounds etc that we came across.

To begin with I went out with my CPT, so I could be introduced to her patients, and have a chance to orientate myself to a different way of working. Once I started seeing people on my own it seemed very isolating, with no one to immediately turn to as on the ward. When I trained as a DN there were no mobile phones, so we had to ask the patients if it was OK to use their house phone, or find a pay phone. This could create a great deal of hanging around, waiting for people such as the doctor to phone back. Mobile phones were finally issued to community nurses a few years later, and to this day is a piece of equipment that revolutionised community service. No longer was it necessary to wait for a call in the patient's home, while time ticked away, and the messaging facility allowed calls to be dealt with when convenient, including from the car.

One of the patients I started seeing became the subject for my patient case study, a major piece of work for the course. Olga, well into her eighties lived in a large detached house in leafy Tilehurst. Her sight was very poor, and registered as blind it was clear she struggled to cope with her home. The grubby kitchen and the un-vacuumed or dusted house drew testimony to this. Most of her time she spent in a room next to the kitchen, probably the breakfast room, and this is where we treated her. Many years before, ring worm in her scalp had been irradiated in

France with large doses of radiotherapy. The result was a chronic wound that penetrated right through her scull, to reveal the dura of her brain. Round the edge of the wound the raw edges were terribly painful, and in consequence difficult to dress. My CPT had tried all sorts, and eventually resorted to simple paraffin gauze. I added an anaesthetic gel to try and relieve the pain at dressing change. It helped a bit but stung when first applied. Olga keen on yoga, used to say everything had: "A cause and effect", and she was right. Once the dressing was in place Olga liked her grey wig that resembled a dead hamster put over the top. When Olga eventually moved into a nursing home, her house went to a developer who did it up, and built a second house of equal size in the garden, two sumptuous family homes

Supervised Practice, where each student in effect worked as a qualified DNS, with supervision, happened at a different surgery. I went to Theale Surgery a large mainly rural practice, different from the urban population nursed at Grovelands, in that the distance covered much increased. The surgery is now Theale Medical Centre, a purpose built facility next to the Old Rectory, and a far cry from the semi detached on the Bath Road where I trained. The house bulged at the seams, with a tiny waiting room, and consulting rooms in every nook and cranny. Our room, on the half landing with creaking stairs, had been converted from a large cupboard, very cosy when all four of us met up. Some of our equipment was kept in the old coach house in the back garden. All the staff were a cheerful bunch, and very supportive of student DNs, I never felt unable to ask silly questions, and despite being very busy everyone from those in the DN team, doctors and receptionists had time for me.

My caseload of patients for the placement had a broad range of conditions to give me the experience required. They gave me the chance to demonstrate to my mentor at the surgery, and my CPT that I could make the right treatment decisions, and prioritise the work according to need. Daily insulins, leg ulcers, terminal illness, catheters, suture and clip removal,I had them all. This differed from hospital where each ward had its own speciality, on the community we looked after everything. Leg ulcers in community nursing are common place, and though I had come across them as an "optional extra", I knew very little about the management of these chronic wounds and that a patient may have them many years.

Elsie was my leg ulcer patient, she lived in a tiny semi, two up two down, with her small elderly husband. Both her legs, badly ulcerated, originally had minor wounds that failed to heal after six weeks, when they officially become leg ulcers. Due to venous insufficiency where the valves on the return veins are damaged, they deteriorated, and twenty five years on, despite everyone's best efforts the ulcers on both legs were extensive, wet and smelly. The weather was hot, and they needed dressing everyday, for despite compression bandages, to support circulation, the bandages were soaked through in twenty four hours. On this particular morning I sat Elsie in the small hot front room, and proceeded to remove the dressings. As I reached the final layer I thought I saw something move, and as I lifted the dressing several big fat maggots dropped out. Mesmerised for a second, I promptly grabbed the plastic rubbish bag, scooped them all up and tightly tide the top. Luckily Elsie, whose sight was poor didn't notice, and the maggots had made a good unorthodox job of cleaning the wound. I recounted the morning to my nursing colleagues, and said I needed a gin and tonic.

My mentor introduced me to a Lord and Lady who had fallen on hard times, and moved into an apartment on a relative's country estate. The apartment opened straight onto the garden and had a calm atmosphere. To compound their situation, he had motor neurone disease, with a short prognosis. They were both very matter of fact about it, and determined to keep a stiff upper lip. When I visited one day, her Ladyship announced that this "thing" had been delivered, and could I show them what to do with it. This turned out to be a portable suction machine, used for clearing oral secretions. They had had the suction machine sometime, and when opened the lid I found mouse droppings inside. They both thought this was frightfully funny, and declared they were not surprised, as there were plenty of mice in the flat.

At the time of my supervised practice some patients still received personal care from the DN team. Historically patients had been bathed and got up by a DNS, though many had a home help instead. Joan who had had a stroke received a weekly bath, this took up most of the morning, as she had a walk in tub, that had to be filled once she was in it. When the wash finished, all the water had to be drained away before Joan got out, and then the tub had to be cleaned.

The other person I saw, in her early thirties with two young children, had debilitating multiple sclerosis. If we attended her for catheter care, on those days it meant getting her washed and downstairs. The stairs, steep and narrow, became more problematical for both her and the nurse helping her down. We both nearly landed in a heap at the bottom one morning, unsafe for both her and me. I called a case conference with her physiotherapist and occupational therapist, and had her care reviewed. With her agreement the bed came downstairs, and a full care package set up.

Personal care moved from medical care, to social care, as a trained nurse is not needed to get someone up and dressed. The problem being that medical care is free, and social care is means tested, and it proved hard to change some of the last few patients over, as they did not want to pay. When I started a new post at Grovelands I was not popular with two patients on my inherited caseload, as I stopped the DN service, and handed them over to social service carers. This freed up nursing time for nursing duties, that have increased year on year. A new saying came about directed at nurses: "Too posh to wash". These people did not realise all the skilled duties a trained nurse should do, and that any nurse would willingly show carers what to do, or wash an incontinent patient if the need arose.

For the experience of different neighbourhoods I did a couple of shifts in the densely populated, working class area of Whitley. An Asian family I visited lived in a damp, dirty terrace. They were very polite, and when I asked for a hand towel he went to take off the none too clean turban from his head, then smiled and thought better of it, producing a rag from elsewhere.

Being unfamiliar with the area, I managed to visit the wrong house one day. I either had the right house number and the wrong street or vice versa. The door when I knocked swung open, so it looked as though I was expected. I called out the person's name, and he responded. I introduced myself and said his daughter had asked me to visit about his dressing. He replied that he didn't have a daughter or a dressing, though he had replied to the name I had used. Realising I had come to the wrong place I apologised and extracted myself quickly, as no one at base would have a clue where I had got to. The only other time I felt vulnerable was later in my career, when I visited an elderly man in an isolated house, whose son shut and double locked the front door in a narrow passage as soon as I entered. In fact they were both polite and friendly, but it was one of those goose bump moments.

Towards the end of Supervised Practice, we had to work over a weekend alone, though we did have a contact number for the DNS in the next patch. On the Friday afternoon I took down all the details for patients from Theale, Mortimer and Pangbourn Surgery, as one DN covered these surgeries at a weekend. The list was lengthy, with details such as: Rose Cottage with large hedge three gates up from oak tree on corner. I started early on Saturday morning, with my visits at Theale, then worked my way round a huge mainly rural patch. My bleep went three times, Reddock, the on call doctor's service (now Westcall), needed a DN to see patients that had rung in that day. With no mobile phones this relied on the good will of a patient to let me use their phone, as the surgeries were shut at the weekend. My list got longer and longer. Some of the patients that had been handed over did not need a visit at all, two I went to needed cream applied, and proved more than capable of applying the medicament themselves. I ended up with twenty one visits, and didn't finish until six pm. On Sunday I had a few less, it turned out to be the busiest weekend I ever worked.

After final exams at the end of the course, everyone

in the set anxiously waited to see what jobs would be available, to start in September. There was no annual leave for the duration of the course, the whole entitlement was taken in August. With added good weather we took the children boating on a wonderful extended trip. On return, I had past my Diploma in Community Nursing and Health, and my new neighbourhood manager (now nurse manager) offered me a district nursing sister's post, four days a week at Circuit Lane Surgery.

Chapter 12: The Virtual Ward

At Circuit Lane Surgery, the DN team had a room at the local clinic in Coronation Square, as the surgery didn't have a spare room. On my first morning, dressed in my navy blue dress with white piping on the collar, I met up with W, the DNS. W had been a DN for years, and had been with Circuit Lane Surgery for a long time. We headed out together so I could start meeting the patients, and familiarise myself with the daily routine. First a quick trip to the surgery to pick up any messages in the DN book, then diabetics for insulin injections, dressings, blood tests, terminal care and so on. After each person had completed their morning visits we met up for lunch, with team members to discuss any issues that arose that morning. We also completed nursing records, and responded to further visits that had to be seen that day. I settled in to my new role, and with W's help started to find my feet.

It took me a while to adapt fully to community nursing, and get better at managing time when the "ward" was spread out in people's houses. On a hospital ward a quick nip to the treatment room, and all that I needed was at hand. In the community this equivalent meant going back to base and out again, my boot stock increased. Procedures had to be tailored to the community too. I had a patient who had a post operative packing to be removed. In hospital intramuscular pethidine would be given prior to the procedure. In the community this took me the whole morning to arrange. I got a prescription from the doctor, dropped it at the patient's house for a relative to get the drug from a chemist, then he phoned me so I could go and give the injection. Then I had to wait for the pethidine to take effect, and finally remove the packing and dress the wound. After that, and I could see W smiling to herself, I rang the patient to ask them to take two paracetamol prior to my visit in about half an hour.

In my early days of district nursing, there was no policy as such, for pet control when they lived with a patient. This meant that some patients saw no problem with their pets being present while I visited. I could ask for the animal to be shut out of the room for cross infection measures, and most patients were fine with this, but not all. On my hands and knees, burrowing round a large pair of legs as I dressed them, I found myself trying to clean the nose of an inquisitive Jack Russell, ensconced under the chair. At another patient I had just got my sterile dressing pack carefully laid out, when a large tabby cat sailed through the air from the sideboard, and landed smack in the middle of it, and I had to start all over again. Chummy, a terrier, and Tibbles the cat would spend an entire visit having a play fight, wrestling with each other, while growling and hissing. Their owner cheerfully chatted away, completely unconcerned, while I could hardly hear myself think. These incidents had never happened on a hospital ward!. In later years, part of the agreement for us to see a patient changed and treatment withdrawn if pets were not properly controlled, withdrawal rarely happened.

There was a small army of people, men and women who had a urinary catheter, to manage a range of bladder problems in the community Like a train spotter who knew all the trains, I could recite chapter and verse size type and make of catheters, drainage bags and accessories. The bags came in three hundred and fifty, five hundred and seven hundred and fifty millilitres, with a direct, short or long inlet tube, and lever or barrel emptying tap. A drainage bag could be attached to the leg with straps, net sleeves, or a sporran belt round the waist. To reduce the risk of the catheter being pulled a g-strap round the leg, or waist to support a supra-pubic catheter were available. At night a two litre overnight drainage bag would be joined at the outlet tap to increase capacity. The night bag had to be rinsed through and hung up to drain, and replaced once a week. This was identified as an infection risk, and later these drainable bags were replaced by a one use new bag every night.

This plumbing may sound complicated, and it was for elderly patients who fumbled with the equipment, wrestled with the emptying tap and generally got into difficulties. For some it was an impossibility to use a no touch technique to reduce risk of urinary tract infection, at the weekly change of their leg bag, and for these patients the HCA visited to do this for them. I had an elderly man who, if in the middle of his wash, didn't bother to put anything on, as he was afraid he would not get to the door in time. Unperturbed he flung the door open, stark naked apart from his sporran bag swinging from his waist. I pointed out to him it was lucky it was me, and not the postman, to which he responded he was sure it was me.

A long term catheter lasted up to three months before it had to be changed, and some patients had a catheter for years. They were used to the procedure, as the old catheter would be removed, and the anaesthetic gel inserted. With men, to stop the gel coming straight out, the tip of the penis had to be squeezed shut by the nurse. Without the slightest embarrassment on either part, I held the penis, and we would chat away about all sorts of subjects, while the gel took effect, before the new catheter could be inserted. All in a day's work.

An interesting visit arose when I had a call to do a joint visit with the Sensory Needs team (SN team). They had a patient who needed short term eye drops for infection, and needed DN input. The patient, deaf dumb and blind required special communication, so that he understood the DN was there for his drops. With no sensory perception except feel, he relied on the SNs team to sign to him, on his hand as he had no sight. Without concept of day or night, he had a sensory clock that he felt to tell the time, deaf and dumb from birth, he lost his sight later in life. On a subsequent visit I let myself in, and touched him on the shoulder as I had been shown to let him know I was there to do his drops. He mistook me for one of his SNs team, and started signing. I took his hand and laid my fingers in a letter "V", to indicate who I was, and touched his cheek. He raised his head and smiled, realising his mistake.

My neighbourhood manager knew I wanted full time work, so she offered me a one day a week secondment to train social service carers. I could fit this in round my DN work, so usually taught each afternoon at Parkside Residential Home. This was an early cross working initiative, aimed at up-skilling care assistants, so they would be able to catch problems such as a developing pressure sore, and alert the DN service earlier rather than later for treatment. Keen to learn, I found the best way to organise the lesson would be to use a flip chart, hung up on the back of a commode, independent of temperamental projectors. On the last session we had a quiz with prizes for all the staff together. Parkside, along with Alice Burrows and Edward Hughes residential homes, purpose built in the 1970s, all closed before 2011, and bull-dozed to the ground. Two are now housing estates, and Alice Burrows, a demolition site, yet to become Alice Burrows Close.

By this time Charlie and Georgette had both started school, and a permanent full time post became available at Grovelands Medical Centre, where I had had my practical placement in training. I suppose all parents who both work full time, wonder what effect it has on their children. Charlie went through an awkward stage when he was little, and Georgette in her teens, this may have happened if I had not worked, who knows. Both have ended up with an excellent work ethic. The plus side of course, that we could afford to go on holiday, and long distance for special occasions. The four of us went to America for my fortieth, and New Zealand for our twenty fifth wedding anniversary, we hired a motorhome to tour these stunning countries.

At the interview for the Grovelands post, my neighbourhood manager, my colleague and one of the surgery doctors interviewed me. I remember him asking me if the travelling would be a problem. I said with a straight face it would double the distance, and take ten minutes to get to work, instead of five. The post was offered to me and I accepted.

I settled in with my new colleagues, and with the surgery team. Everything communication wise, that little bit easier than working for Circuit Lane, as the DN room and storeroom was in the surgery building and not separate. Doctors popped their heads round the door at coffee time, when they all came out of morning surgery, and the doctors employed Hazel who made everyone a hot drink- luxury. We had a lot of fun, and sometimes they came to see what the laughter was about. The DNs could nip along and hover outside the door if something required the doctor. However the wait could be prolonged, and this we referred to as "camping out", with people passing who would remark we were still waiting. Most Doctors I have come across are very good about being available, despite being in the middle of a list of patients. They realise that without that prescription, or piece of advice they held up our work, and the timely treatment of, for example a poorly patient needing drug adjustment for the syringe driver.

The visits on my caseload were varied and interesting, with the usual range of district nursing duties. I had a request to see a lady to advise about wound management. Val, in her fifties had hidradenitis suppurativa, a condition where boils form on the lymph glands in the axillae. The wounds were painful and constantly leaked on to her clothes, Val took high doses of morphine for the pain, and said she had been told nothing more could be done, and she would have to manage. On inspection there appeared a deep pocket under her arm, full of putrid pus, and a bridge of skin that made cleaning very difficult. After some thought we found the best way to clean the pocket, was to get Val to lean over the bath, then I irrigated with a large syringe to flush the puss out, and packed the wound with Kaltostat, a seaweed packing. I also asked the doctor to refer her to the dermatologist, the skin bridge once removed made wound toilet easier.

I knew Val had an ulcer on her leg, that she self managed. When I looked at this wound, it covered an area of about ten by ten centimetres, with smelly slough. Val and I decided that this could do with daily cleansing. Doppler ultrasound, where the venous circulation is measured with a hand held probe denoted that Val would be suitable for reduced compression bandaging, and once this took effect we reduced the leg dressing to twice and then once weekly. With antibiotics, improved management of her insulin dependent diabetes, and treatment of anaemia with ferrous sulphate (iron) tablets, the wounds improved. I gradually reduced the morphine, and Val stopped taking it. Her husband doted on her, he was one of those people that liked to put medical people on the spot. Any new medication and out would come his MIMS, one of the drug information books we used, and I would be quizzed on all the side effects. Sometime after I had finished seeing Val, John had a myocardial infarction and died, no surprise as he smoked heavily and had hypertension despite his interest in health

A patient of my colleague's, like John died mainly due to the choices she had made regarding her health. Betty lived with her husband John, who because of her morbid obesity acted as her main carer. Though totally blind he did everything from washing Betty, meal preparation and shopping, escorted by his guide dog for the blind. In the house it was incredible to see him move around, he knew every inch, and watching him you could not tell he saw nothing. Betty had leg ulcers, and decreasing mobility, and because of this took to her bed where she developed a bed sore. We could get a commode to put by the bed, but in this instance social services went through a stage of issuing a camping Porta-Potti instead. These are not very big, and poor Betty enveloped it like a mother hen sitting on an egg, and then struggled to get up

This type of toilet comes in two sections, a tank surrounding the bowl has the flush water, and the lower tank is for the sewage. No thought seemed to have gone as to who, or where it should be emptied. Ideally a low open drain is needed to empty the sewage, as the cassette is heavy, and the contents easily splashed when poured out. Emptying into a normal toilet is awkward, and these chemical toilets were not issued for long. Betty's decreased mobility in bed meant her legs were raised, and stopped weeping, but her overall health deteriorated and she died. Because of her size she had the bed in the front room of their tiny terrace. The undertaker found it impossible to get her body out of the room, so called the Fire Brigade. They removed the sash window, frame and all, and extracted her through the window and over the garden wall.

With an interest in how people live, I had the opportunity to get to know people, and their houses very well, as some patients would be on the caseload for years. Several had houses that were like stepping back in time as I entered the front door. One lady lived opposite the old Reading Football Stadium (now houses), and once through the front door of her terrace house, I could have been in the 1940's. The umbrella and cloak stand stood in the narrow hall, with its moulded plaster arch, and dark brown doors leading off to the front and back rooms, the stairs with a runner and brass stair rods ran up straight ahead. All the furniture had been purchased new when Jean got married, and had been all the vogue, the retro three piece suite was deep seated, with curved arms and beige material. The dining room table had a lace cloth, as did the radio where the cat rested. The power points, were still the old fashioned three pin type, and meant I had to find an adaptor for my machine in order to syringe her ears. The telephone, made of bakelite, with a proper dial, was the last one I came across of this type.

In a street running down to the Oxford road two elderly spinster sisters lived, then one remained on her own. My colleague visited one day and got no reply, I went round for moral support as we did not know why there was no reply. We let ourselves in, calling her name, and searching through the house incase she lay unconscious. The three story townhouse had lots of rooms, with Edwardian furniture and decoration. There were no modern appliances, an o-so-cool in the pantry, and a solid fuel range plus ancient Flaval gas cooker in the kitchen. No reply came to our calls, and it transpired the lady had been admitted to hospital.

Some patients were hoarders, of objects or rubbish. I called at a large house on the Tilehurst road, to find the door ajar, so I called out, and he said to come through. The whole house appeared to be full of newspapers, stacked thigh high with a narrow passage to squeeze through. The papers lined the hall, went up the stairs, and surrounded him in his front room. As I walked in he quoted the old rhyme: "Light me a candle to take me to bed, and fetch me a chopper to chop off your head", a bit disconcerting to say the least. Thankfully I did not need to go back. A man in The Birds Mobile Home Park had so much rubbish in his home a space had to be cleared to make enough room for me and the dressing pack that had to rest on more rubbish.

In Sherwood Street a lady who had very wet leg ulcers lived with her husband and daughter. The front room in hot weather had a strong smell of pseudomonas. (Pseudomonas is a bacterium that can infect and colonise wounds, and smells like bad onions). In an effort to keep up appearances Joan decided to buy a new three piece suite, when it came it dwarfed the room, and blocked the way in and out up the stairs. Joan phoned the firm and demanded that it be collected, claiming they had not told her how big it was. Reluctantly they came, I wonder if they ever got rid of the smell from that room, so the suite could be sold on.

In Armatige Road I had a northern European lady, with a very forceful daughter. Seldom would a day go by, that she did not phone me or social services. If the call came to me, it would be regarding her mother's continence pads. However hard I tried to get the type and delivery sorted out, things were never quite right. I did wonder if mother was in fact entitled to this service, and I am afraid I shrank from bringing the subject up, as to whether she had British citizenship. The other problem was that mother's mobility had deteriorated, and the semi-detached house, situated on a bank had three flights of steps to the front door. Despite the handrails all the way up, the poor lady took longer and longer to climb them, and became virtually wheelchair bound. After a lot of negotiation the daughter acquired a garden lift. The lift was supplied and funded, to the tune of around ten thousand pounds by social services. The lift required extensive earth removal to install, and equalled something that would not have looked out of place at Alton Towers, when it was finally finished. By this time things had moved on, it broke down on both occasions the daughter used it for her mother, who then went into a home anyway, as the daughter could no longer manage her at home. Then the discussion started as to who should take the lift away, as it de-valued the house. Despite all this I had to admire those two, the daughter would drive her mother on the long journey back home to the continent, in their ageing Vauxhall Cavalier that I would not have trusted as far as the local shops.

"The hills are alive to the sound of music", echoed

through my mind as I recall the Carmelite Monastery in Southcote Lane. The clang of the door bell echoed deep in the house, and after a pause I'd hear the swish of the nun's habit on the flag stones. Her face would appear in a small aperture in the door, framed by her white head piece, accompanied by a lovely smile. This was a fascinating insight into a closed order of nuns, who only went out for medical purposes, (of which there were quite a number), and had few visitors. Mother superior would then escort me through the house and upstairs, past other nuns at work. Their day started early at four am with prayers, work and breakfast at eight o'clock. Then more work, making rice paper discs for communion, which gave them a small income. Followed by lunch, prayers, and a rest period where they listened avidly to the radio, (no television), and did sewing, supper, prayers and bed by ten, ready for next day. Around twelve of then lived there, mother superior worried as the numbers dropped that no new novices were forthcoming. They only had one novice, a sweet Irish girl of twenty one, I wondered how she had decided on this course of life, at such a young age in this day and age.

Because of their commitment to God, and secluded lifestyle, they were very interested in what went on in the outside world, and bent over backwards to make visitors feel welcome. The bedrooms upstairs, were simply furnished with a single bed that overlooked the garden from a sash window. The bedrooms varied from large and spacious, to a box room size as the house was Victorian. My favourite bit, the provision for hand washing. On the table by the window two china jugs stood, one with hot water, one with cold, a china basin, soap on a white enamel dish, and a pressed linen towel would be ready. With anticipation I would wait for the attending nun to pour the water from each jug into the basin to just the right temperature for my hands, and stand ready with the hand towel. Hand washing to a whole new level. All the nuns were very caring, and one would sit with a poorly member day and night. I visited one day and the novice had been gently rubbing a necrotic (dead) toe for hours while praying that life would return to the affected digit.

In the end the Catholic church announced the monastery would close due to lack of numbers, and the nuns would amalgamate with a different convent. Our team at Grovelands were very sorry to see them go. I suggested to mother superior if I bought some buns, and they supply tea, we could say goodbye. We had a lovely tea party, and were shown round their wonderful garden, complete with vegetables, fruit, flowers and lawns. All gone under multiple flats, and the old main house and chapel is almost unrecognisable, even the carriage sweep to the majestic front door disappeared under a car park.

While on the subject of religion, I had a thought provoking visit that widened my horizon. We took it in turns to answer the bleep and take messages, and a lady contacted me to say she didn't know what to do, as she was unable to get her husband off the floor. After a look at his medical notes I found he had been diagnosed with a malignant glioma, a type of brain tumour, pressing on the optic nerve. When I got there he had been unable to get off the ground for three days, one eye bulged like that of Cyclops. He had been working in the Far East and come home briefly to England, and planned to go to the States with his wife and two children, for a new contract. I called the doctor in and ascertained the man did not want to go to hospital, and wished to have his symptoms treated at home with a syringe driver.

I collected the Graseby syringe driver from the surgery, and his wife collected the medication from the chemist. Sitting at the kitchen table I prepared everything on a tray, drew up the drugs, noted the details, and wrote up the notes. Most nurses including me will ask not to be disturbed while the drugs are prepared, as the situation can be tense, and no mistake must be made. Once set up he could receive medication at a continuous rate over twenty four hours, via a fine butterfly needle, that I placed in his upper arm. The Graseby syringe driver, later superseded by the McKinley syringe pump, and pre-emptive drugs are now kept in the house of a patient with terminal illness, so there is no delay in symptom treatment. The usual "in case" drugs were: morphine for pain and breathlessness, metoclopramide for nausea, haloperidol and or midazolam for agitation, and hyocine for excess secretions. In this man's case the syringe driver had to be started on the first visit, so these would not have been available anyway.

The rest of the day, I implored Medical Loans to urgently deliver the bed, pressure relief mattress, hoist, and commode so the gentleman could have his wish and be nursed at home.

Understandably it was a dreadful time for this family, to look after a very sick loved one, who they would soon lose, when they should have been on their way to America. His lovely wife asked me on a subsequent visit, what the family should do about a funeral, as they did not believe in God. I had been brought up in a Church of England family, and though not particularly religious, had not met any atheists. A bit taken aback, I realised that as non believers they were kind people, with values the same as mine, who didn't need God. I had no experience of a non Christian funeral, so asked the Macmillan Nursing Service, who helped the family arrange a celebration of his life.

I had made a joint visit to a man in a ground floor flat in Southcote,very debilitated with heart failure. At the joint visit with his GP, he became adamant that he did not want to be admitted to hospital. All I could do was make him as comfortable as possible, with a rug over his knees, and a hot flask of tea by his side. There I left him next to the fire, surrounded by his beloved collection of musical and war film videos. Next day I returned and got no reply when I rang the bell. Peering through the window I saw him sitting in his chair, there was no movement and I knew he had died. I worked my way round the back of the flats, and climbed in through the kitchen window, and sure enough my fears were confirmed. He sat where I had left him, with a gentle smile on his ashen face. I am sure he knew he would die, and wanted to be at home, he had his wish. The doctor and the ambulance that I had alerted came, and we all agreed resuscitation would not be appropriate, and with no family, the undertaker took over.

In the community it was unusual to be present when a patient died, unless I happened to be visiting at that moment. There were two times when this did occur, one an older and the other a young patient. The elderly gentleman was dying of heart failure, and could be made most comfortable sitting in his chair. On my visit the next morning his limbs showed the mottling that preceded death, with the help of his family we just got him comfortable in bed, where he had asked to go, and he gave a little sigh and was gone.

The other was a young man with terminal illness dying at home. He had a syringe pump with a complicated drug regime running for symptom control that I had just recharged. I looked round after concentrating on my task, and realised he was about to die, his wife came up and he slipped away. The procedure for a death at home is different from hospital, because apart from getting the person tidy, they are left for the undertaker to collect and lay out. Usually the face is not covered at home, unless the family request it.

There was the inventive that verged on the Heath Robinson. Vera lived with her husband Dennis, and a very bumptious Labrador who had never been taught how to behave. The house smelt of dog, and when I knocked on the door I could rely on standing there ten minutes while Dennis bawled at Jessie as he barricaded her into the kitchen. If he had any worries about the dog he asked me about it because I was a nurse and had a dog, so assumed I would know. Vera, wheelchair bound was looked after mainly by Dennis, who always tried to think of things to help his wife. The best invention he made consisted of a shoe box on a pulley system he had tied from head to foot rail of the hospital bed. This enabled Vera to keep the phone, channel changer etc safe at the bottom of the bed for later retrieval without cluttering her bed table.

The unexpected happened at a visit to a man who had recently had a tracheotomy to assist breathing due to throat cancer. He was elderly and despite the amount of sputum he produced, gamely tried to manage his trachy tube. We were in the bathroom and he momentarily loosened his grip and coughed, as I tied the retaining tapes at the back of his neck. The tube shot straight out and arched gracefully onto the floor. With no time to do anything else as he spluttered and choked, I rinsed it hastily under the tap and re-inserted the silver tube back into the opening in his neck, prior to exchange for a sterile tube.

Time off and holidays was something everyone and that included me, looked forward too. They were an essential part of work, as we all needed to recharge our batteries, to be able to remain fresh and effective at work. I always tried, as did others to have a quiet afternoon prior to annual leave, and get away in good time. Occasionally this just did not go to plan. My manager rang at lunchtime on a Friday, to say that the Trust had a major care and safety concern at a local nursing home. All DNS's were required to interview the staff and patients of the home, check all the nursing records, and write a report for submission by five o'clock that day. We all duly dropped everything and went to the home. The atmosphere was very tense, as the staff could not be told why we had been sent in, and were stressed and anxious. This took a considerable number of hours, and we were all late home.

The other time this happened to me was later as a CM (Community Matron), with a patient who had alcoholic liver failure. I had only recently met him, and when I visited that Friday I could see he was very poorly, confused and incontinent of liquid diarrhoea. He had been in and out of hospital for treatment, and I asked the family what they had been told about his prognosis while on the ward. It was obvious to me he had become terminal, and further treatment would not have any benefit. I rang the registrar on the ward, and he agreed with me on this point, so I explained to the family he would be best nursed at home if we could manage and arrange this. After helping them to clean him up, I spoke to his GP, who agreed home management would be sensible. For the rest of the day I arranged delivery of the equipment he needed, made sure he had appropriate medication for symptom control, spoke to rapid response to start personal care that day, set up Marie Curie nursing service for the night, and asked the DN on at the weekend to visit. The family were very grateful for all the time I had given them, and I went on holiday with the buzz of a great sense of satisfaction in a job well done.

Chapter 13: Leg Ulcers and District Nursing

A large part of a district nursing caseload is taken up with the treatment and management of leg ulcers. Simplistically, a wound is counted as a leg ulcer if it is on the lower leg and has not healed within six weeks. There are three types, venous, arterial and mixed (venous and arterial). Venous ulcers occur when the vein valves are damaged, and blood fluids back flow into the tissues. Arterial ulcers occur when the arteries narrow, and there is reduced blood supply to the legs. Mixed ulcers are a combination of both. Venous ulcers are commonest, and about three quarters of them can be successfully healed with compression bandage therapy, pioneered by the nurse Christine Moffat. Ulcers that heal are a satisfying part of nursing, and then there is the quarter that don't heal, and take up a lot of time. The reasons for these non-healing ulcers are many. Other co-morbidities (illnesses) like diabetes, renal failure, and obesity can all reduce healing rate, along with low compliance with the treatment, and lifestyle choices that are derogatory to healing, poor diet, smoking, and lack of exercise.

I tried wearing compression bandages for a day, in order to understand why, even when the benefits are explained, patients may well decide they did not want the bandages as they felt tight and restrictive. My bandages did feel tight and restrictive, though I decided this preferable to a leg with a wet smelly unhealed ulcer. The bandage systems we used were either four, three or two layer. Four layer consisted of Sofban (synthetic wool) for comfort absorption and leg shaping, a crepe bandage to hold the wool, and keep the desired leg shape of graduated widening ankle to knee, then an elastic bandage , and finally, an adhesive outer layer, both applied with fifty percent stretch to achieve the correct compression. If the Doppler denoted a mixed ulcer, the third layer, the elasticated bandage would be omitted. In mixed ulcers with slight arterial blockage compression is reduced, as the circulation must not be stopped, (the reason why compression is never used on limbs with severe arterial occlusion). The two layer bandage system achieved the same compression as four, in a slightly different way, and consisted of wool, and a short stretch non elastic outer bandage applied at a hundred percent stretch. The leg would then be redressed weekly, and more often if the wound leaked copious fluid.

In a patient who I wanted to start compression therapy with, preparatory work prior to bandage application went a long way to acceptance. It would not be just the bandages that the patient had to accept, but also changes to bad habits of a lifetime in regards to diet, exercise, and smoking cessation. They would also need to wear compression stockings to stop recurrence of the ulcer, forever once the wounds healed. Despite the best efforts of any treating nurse, bandages might be fiddled with. It was not unknown for a patient to stick a knitting needle down the inside of the bandage to scratch at an itch, causing more skin damage, or even the entire removal of bandage and dressing.

A joint visit with the doctor for moral support, when everything had been tried to encourage the person to have the correct treatment could be useful. An elderly man I had on the Oxford Road lived in a cold stark house, where the kitchen tap had leaked so badly and so long, the water had rotted the floor as it splashed out of the sink. When I returned on my second visit, the bandages on his leg had vanished, and he denied all knowledge of them. Eventually I tracked the bandages down under the sideboard, chopped into tiny pieces with a pair of scissors. This happened on the next visit despite protracted discussion and his agreement to try again. With the support of the doctor, he had to be sectioned under the Mental Health Act for psychiatric treatment, as he had become completely divorced from reality.

I went on a joint visit with the doctor, to a lady of mine who had mixed ulcers, steadily decreasing mobility and inability to cope at home. Each visit I discussed with her and her husband their options for care, all politely declined. With the doctor at the visit things came to a head, when her husband announced in so many words that they could no longer manage. He, a retired Reading Abattoir slaughter man, with a broad Berkshire accent, drew himself up, and holding onto the back of the sofa announced: "me 'ip's gorn, an I'm completely buggered". It summed the whole situation up perfectly, and they agreed to our suggestions.

Marg, a patient that had non healing ulcers, took up a large amount of our team's time. Marg had transferred to Grovelands from a local surgery, as she had moved in with her daughter and grandson, complete with her ulcers of twenty five years standing. These ulcers started from small trauma injuries received while gardening, and never healed completely. Over the years the downward spiral of weight gain, poorly controlled diabetes, osteoarthritis, and reduced mobility, lead to extensive wounds on not only both lower legs, but thighs as well. In a case like this, the ulcers realistically will never heal, however the ulcers can usually be better managed, and the accompanying wetness they cause reduced.

I knew my first visit would be a long one, and put plenty of time aside. Marg, very used to having a DN in everyday, had a huge box of dressings, bandages and pads, enough to start a chemist shop. Different nurses had tried one dressing, and moved promptly on to the next when no improvement happened. The problem is the dressing in contact with the wound will make little difference, until the underlying causes are addressed. Talking to Marg about her diet, glucose and weight control were like water off a duck's back, she had heard it all before, and nodded patiently, while I went through it again.

Once I had checked her circulation with the doppler, Marg agreed to try short stretch (two layer compression) again, that she had had in the past. This in itself was a mammoth task, both legs in total required twelve Mepitel contact dressings, twelve large absorbent pads, two meters of tubigauze to hold dressing and pads in place, ten synthetic wool, four seven centimetre and four ten centimetre short stretch self adhesive bandages. Initially this had to be changed everyday, as the wetness decreased the dressings were changed every other day, occasionally the dressings lasted three days.

Apart from the time and cost, the whole visit became physically demanding, and resembled a work out at the gym. I decided to split the visit in half, so our health care assistant would go in first, strip the bandages and dressings, wash the legs in a bowl of water, make a list of supplies to reorder, and ring me. I would be at a visit near by, to go round as soon as I could, so the wounds were not exposed too long. Then all the dressings and bandages had to be replaced. The only way to place the Mepitel, on the back of the thighs, was to ask Marg to stand up and turn round, so I could see where to place them. This took Marg sometime, as true to form of those with reduced mobility, her large armchair had a tide of possessions that cascaded from it, further hampering her standing up, and my ability to get in a good position to dress the legs. I used to kneel on the floor, sweating in my plastic apron, as I rhythmically rocked to and fro applying the layers of bandages, toe to groin. Her calf measured the same as my waist, to give an idea of proportion.

Millie had a non healing arterial ulcers and both legs were swollen and wet due to her heart failure, diabetic neuropathy meant her feet and hands had no feeling, and diabetic retinopathy rendered her almost blind. I had worked hard to get her a little less dependent on our service, and had spent a lengthy visit with the diabetes nurse specialist, trying to teach Millie how to use an Innolet insulin injection device. This had a large dial like an egg timer with big numbers, plus an audible click to count up the correct dose of insulin. Although Millie managed this after a fashion, she could not un-screw and change the needle without pricking her fingers, and nurses were not allowed to do this due to the risk of needle stick injury. (Later a self sheathing needle came onto the market that would have solved this problem). Millie became a daily visit to give her insulin, and dress her legs.

When she had been more mobile she had attended the surgery for dressings, and would turn up with sticky polish homemade treats, very kind, but the cat hair was off putting, and they ended up in the bin. Her husband died, her mobility decreased, and the heart failure worsened. She collapsed on my visit one day, and necessitated a 999 call, Millie survived, and came home from hospital before her final admission when she died. In among all the commotion my coat, over a chair got too close to the gas fire, with a horrible smell of singeing, luckily I noticed in time before real damage occurred.

Ted lived just up the road from the surgery, and like Millie initially came to the surgery for leg ulcer dressing before he became housebound. He drove the two hundred yards in his green Mark 1 Escort, which was old and dented on every panel. If we were in the office there would be no need to look out of the window, as his visit would be heralded by the tortured scream of gearbox and clutch as he manoeuvred. Anyone who thought their car might be in range hastily stopped what they were doing and ran out to move their vehicle out of the way. He was known to everyone as Clutch Slip Ted.

In a large faded townhouse on the corner of Argyle Street, with the garden overrun with brambles lived Marjorie. Nothing had changed since her husband had died of a heart attack in their kitchen. His car, a 1970s eighteen hundred sat unused in the garage, keys in the ignition as if he intended to nip out. The lodgers they had had upstairs had gone, Marjorie locked the door at the top of the stairs, and never went up there again. I would visit in the afternoon, as Marjorie did not get up before about one o'clock, and stayed up late into the night. She had a few friends, but her outings and contacts slowly petered out. I knew she would be alone for Christmas, and organised for the Salvation Army to pick her up for their Christmas Lunch. Marjorie, keen on the idea at the time, declined to go when they came for her. The small ulcer on her stick like leg eventually healed. Normally I would have discharged her. Marjorie made out all was fine. Yet I knew she hardly ate anything, her neat crimperlene slacks and top remained unchanged, her fridge had stopped working, and that I was the one person she saw from one week to the next. Her only elderly relative lived miles away, and Marjorie had no one. The mental health team took her over once her dementia became confirmed, and Marjorie eventually went to a nursing home close to her sole relative.

The time that a leg ulcer visit took gave the advantage of time to chat to the person while dressing the legs. Two patients had been brought up in Reading remembered horse drawn vehicles when they were used everyday, and as I drive a pony and trap myself, I found these accounts particularly fascinating. John, who had been a green grocer said his horse refused to go under Reading West railway bridge, and he had to resort to going via Little John's Lane, or go up to the Tilehurst Road. I wondered about this, as the bridge is high, and the road wide. Years later I found a picture of the bridge in the 1940s, as it had been, the picture showed a narrow brick tunnel bridge, spooky indeed for some horses, especially if a steam train ran over the top. John said a loose bolting horse and cart was a relatively common sight, a dangerous situation as the frightened animal will gallop through or over anything, cart and all. I think that this occurred because there were more horse drawn vehicles, and the breaking (training) of horse to cart, possibly rushed in the need of a new driving animal. Mary reported that a horse bolted near her home, in Beresford Road, and the shafts ended up jammed through the railing, inches from her baby's head in his pram. John and Mary both chatted about the small stable yards at the back of some of the terrace houses near the Oxford Road. They were accessed by an archway through to the back, these can still be seen today, a glimpse of architecture for a bygone era.

On a brighter note to end this chapter, I went to see a security guard in Overdown Road. He had so much pain from his ulcerated legs, his wife did not know what to do with him, as he crawled round the house on his knees. The man lay on his bed and cried out with pain, so I asked the doctor to visit and prescribe analgesia and antibiotics for infection. Once four layer bandages could be applied, he quickly improved. The legs healed, and three months later he went back to work, conscientiously wearing his new compression stockings. A text book example of how ulcers can heal.

Chapter 14:A Young Gentleman of Fragile Disposition

Alongside the steady tide of visits I had training. The Trust like all employers had to provide mandatory training. This included fire procedure, moving and handling, and statutory training specific to the requirements of the job such as resuscitation, influenza vaccination, syringe driver, and central line updates for example. Some were attended yearly, or two yearly, and accounted for around ten days per annum. In addition to this were my own personal development, study days I chose, to keep my practice up to date. This included new research, and meeting up with professionals from different teams, continence, diabetes, dementia, and other disciplines, medics, physiotherapy, and social services to name but a few.

An advantage of working for the NHS is the offer of sponsorship for a degree course that could be tailored round a full time job. I had an inkling that doing a degree would be a wise move. District Nurse training had moved from District Nursing Certificate, to Diploma, to Degree course, and the nurses that ran the Continence service had had to re-apply against each other, as three posts became one. My distance learning Degree in Health and Community Studies had four modules and a dissertation that had to be completed between two and five years. I finished mine in 2004 after two years, and received my first class degree at a wonderful ceremony at Reading

University, complete with cap and gown. Alistair, Mum and Hugh, my brother over from New Zealand came, and we drank celebratory champagne in the garden afterwards.

Two years later I completed my Independent Nurse Prescribing Course. This is when a trained nurse, who has passed the course, and in the right circumstances can prescribe medication. The Cumberlege report had first mooted the idea about ten years earlier, and eventually with the agreement of doctors and pharmacists (who can also be prescribers), the act to allow nurses to prescribe came to fruition. There was a huge amount to get through, and required discipline to come in from work, and sit at the computer for a couple of hours each evening, as I had done for my degree course. Exams included a three hour paper, plus live consultation, and detailed drug portfolio. I felt particularly pleased at gaining this qualification as it proved to be so useful, Very glad I did it when I did, as it has got progressively hard to pass. The drug calculation test that was brought in, required a hundred percent pass mark, maths has never been my strong point, and I don't know if I ever could have achieved that mark. I had my own ways of calculating, and ran the finances at home. I just can't do percentages and problem solving maths.

Removal of a male catheter caused discomfort when the deflated balloon that held the catheter in place, passed down the urethra, I invented a method that I felt should be more comfortable. I wondered if the outgoing catheter could be used to introduce the anaesthetic gel, through the catheter, and out through the drainage eyes from within the bladder, through the urethra and out of the penile meatus (tip). This meant that the gel would help lubricate the catheter as it came out, and lubricate the urethra from inside to out, ready for insertion of the new catheter. To introduce the gel into the penis, the tip of a preloaded syringe is inserted in the urethral meatus (opening), and the plunger firmly depressed. The gel usually spurts out round the side, and may not be as effective as it should be.

 Any research has to go in front of an ethics committee, I applied to do a pilot study of ten patients, had permission granted, and found my sample of patients willing to participate, so the trial began. A urinary catheter is held in the bladder with a ten mil balloon of sterile water, deflated before removal by drawing the water into a syringe from a valve connected to a fine tube, running along side the drainage channel that is incorporated in the catheter. Once this had been done, the catheter bag that collected the urine, would be disconnected from the catheter, and the gel inserted down the drainage tube, while slowly withdrawing the catheter from the urethra. When I had completed the procedure I asked the man a set of questions, for example: "On a scale of nought to ten, nought being no pain, and ten severe pain, how much discomfort did you feel when I removed the catheter?" In a comparison group of ten men who had their catheters removed in the normal way, I asked the same set of questions as the research group, and compared the answers. What struck me about doing research was that it needed the support of a research team, as to set it up, gather and to correlate all the information, took a lot of time. The result of my pilot study suggested that my method helped reduce pain, and it would be worth a full study. I couldn't do a full research on my own, and hope that one day someone will go on from where I left off. Even if someone did do this, and proved my method relieved pain, it is difficult to change practice due to the shear size of the NHS.

A case in point, the excellent research by Rosemary Rodgers into ear syringing. Rosemary concluded that in many ears the application of oil over a period, only served to swell and increase the wax, and syringing may not be needed, with its inherent risk of tympanic membrane (ear drum) perforation. Oil could be used for lubrication only, at the time of wax evacuation, using a Jobson Horne probe, and Noots forceps. The method negated the need to oil before syringing, so also saved time. Necessary wax extraction could be made when the ear was examined, with no need for a second visit to syringe, as this required oil for a few days beforehand. Despite changes made in the trust policy to sanction use of the Rodgers method, Rosemary retired, and a lack of trainers has meant syringing has remained common practice.

Some of the trainers or tutors really knew their subject, and made the sessions interesting, and complicated information sound easy, especially with dry subjects such as policy and procedures. Occasionally they didn't quite come up to expectations. On a health promotion course, the tutor floundered her way through the first half hour, and asked the group how the incidence of teenage pregnancy could be reduced. To lighten the session, quick as a flash my colleague suggested the girls keep their legs together, after a stony silence the tutor continued. I am not sure the tutor had had very much patient contact, as she proclaimed all ills could be amended. Patients that I had seen for months sprang to mind, who had made no change to their life style, despite constant support and reminders. I pointed out to the tutor that there were people completely impervious to health promotion. With that the tutor threw up her hands, said she had had enough, and stormed out. The class looked at each other in amazement, and concluded her usual audience must be student nurses, who she could dazzle with her expertise.

Training was held in a number of locations in West Berkshire, such as Sandleford and Newbury District Hospitals (both replaced by West Berkshire Community Hospital), RBH, Stonham Court in Reading, Dellwood (community beds moved to the new Prospect Park Hospital), and Fairmile Hospital at

South Stoke. Occasionally the venue would be Wexham Park Hospital in Slough in East Berks. My preference for these venues were the ones with an interesting drive, and easy parking at the end. The trip out to Fairmile, was not only a favourite venue for me, it also threw up an unusual surprise, fatuously as it turned out, for a record keeping update. On a walkabout during break, I came across a huge room with around fifty trestle tables, piled two feet high with old patient records. The hospital would shortly relocate to Prospect Park, and I imagine they had all been dug out of an ancient archive, and staff were wondering what to do with them. The records dated back to the early 1900s, and on inspection gave a fascinating insight into mental health treatment back then. One started "a young gentleman of a fragile disposition...", and another "this young women of ill repute..." I do hope these records survived, as they would be invaluable for historic medical research.

Two other training sessions worth a mention were for AIDS (Auto Immune Deficiency Syndrome), and later SARS (Severe Acute Respiratory Syndrome originating from Asian bird flu). In both cases there presented a real risk of a pandemic, and regardless of anything else training for them became a priority. There were all sorts of rumours that circulated about AIDS, as the exact source was unknown. Sexual transfer by monkeys could have been to blame, or even camels. This did seem unlikely, because as I said to the trainer, a step ladder would have been required. SARS, an air borne disease dictated that we all had to be issued with a breathing mask, to be used if we visited a patient, known to have SARS, and happened to be having a nebuliser. That I know of this eventuality never occurred, however the individually fitted, double filtered masks everyone was issued with, proved excellent for home decoration, sanding and painting.

Part of my job as a nurse, was to mentor pre registration students, trained nurses, and to teach patients and carers, on a formal basis and any informal opportunity. For the community placement the students would be allocated to one of us to mentor them on a one to one basis. Our team at Grovelands enjoyed the fresh pair of eyes that a student can bring. We had a vested interest, in that in years to come these would be the nurses looking after us in our dotage, should it be necessary. As a rule of thumb, we liked to feel happy if they were to look after our own elderly relatives. Most student nurses were a pleasure to have, keen, asked appropriate questions, polite, liked by the patients, and passed their placement with out any problem.

Then there were the few that had been able to drift through previous placements, and had not done so well. Because they came to the team on a one to one basis, gaps in their practical work and knowledge soon materialised. The first step would be to get a colleague to take the student out, and invariably they would confirm concerns. Each student had a Community Tutor, who came in so the three of us could sit down, talk things through, and come up with an action plan that had to be achieved by the end of the placement. The meeting often revealed that assignments had been referred (failed), and just passed at a second attempt. I can recall a mature student near the end of her training, who was so busy talking to me on leaving a patient, she shut the door in his face, and didn't realise. Not the only incident. A further student nurse who did not seem to have much nursing knowledge, also required an action plan. On a busy hospital ward, it is too easy for a failing student to stand back, and not get the experience they should gain. In both these cases the students managed their action plan. As a sign off mentor near the end of their training, it was a big responsibility to vouch a student fit to practice as a trained nurse. Passing the action plan, objectively meant, as long as they had not done anything dangerous, they had passed.

Teaching other trained nurses could be fun. Four times a year I had a half hour slot on the two day Promotion of Continence course, run by the nurses of CAS (Continence Advisory Service), with a multiple choice and viva exam on the last day. Those attending had lectures on everything about bladder and bowel management, and I taught about the use and application of rectal suppositories and enemata. To kick off the session I asked the audience how many bisocodyl or glycerine suppositories should be administered. Invariable the answer given, would be two, when the answer should be one, as stated in the BNF (British National Formulary). Two had always been the norm, it was only because I read up in the BNF, that I found this out, an example of how a simple mistake can go unnoticed and to my knowledge, there were no reported cases of harm. I joked that we had all been over dosing on suppositories for years, and that I found having changed my practice, one worked just as well as two.

I went to see a lady in her nineties about her urinary incontinence which troubled her. This is a common complaint, and needed skilled assessment to ascertain the cause, and to decide the treatment. There are different types of incontinence, and a care pathway is used, to help assessment. The initial general assessment ruled out infection, and the symptom profile filled in by the patient, denoted the correct pathway to treatment. Pathways exist for all kinds of assessment, they are thorough, and completed over at least two visits.

Stress incontinence, with weakened pelvic floor muscles, means the bladder neck is not adequately supported. Urine will leak from the bladder with the stress of coughing, exercise, or laughing. In urge incontinence, the bladder is very sensitive, there is an over riding urge to pass urine, and out it comes. Urinary retention may be due to an obstruction, such as an enlarged prostate in men, very uncomfortable, and often referred to by a man as his "prostrate". Or due to neurological damage in diabetes, when a full bladder is not felt, and is so full, the urine will force it's way out with no warning.

The lady I visited had stress incontinence. Treatment for this is an exercise regime for the pelvic floor to tone up the muscles that support the bladder. Rose, very attentive, hung on my every word. I explained to her how the pelvic floor muscles, attached to the pelvic ring, support the bladder bowel and vagina where they exit the body, and they should be trampoline tight and not saggy like a hammock. I explained how she could identify the muscles, by stopping the stream of urine when she sat on the loo, and once she identified the muscles, the exercise of these could be practised anywhere. To emphasise my description of how to tense and hold the muscle in a series of quick and then slow contractions, I clenched my fist to emulate the tensing and relaxation of the pelvic floor. At the end of the session I asked Rose to tell me what she had to do, to check she understood. Rose said: "Well I sit on the loo, and go like this", and proceeded to clench and un-clench her fist!. You can't win them all.

If, after assessment a patient did require pads, information would be given to them regarding pad provision from the CAS. As part of their service CAS provided continence products to cater for the needs of incontinent patients, mainly disposable pads. CAS and I always referred to continence products, rather than incontinence, as continence would be the primary aim, with well managed incontinence being a close, and more realistic second. The supply and delivery of pads depended on how incontinent the patient was, and determined the number and absorption of pads provided.

This ranged from two pads or less when the patients bought their own, to three or more pads in twenty four hours, with absorption up to six hundred millilitres for a night time pad. It would not be unknown for patients to stock pile their pads, one had a whole garage full!. In consequence pads cost the trust a substantial overspend. CAS tackled this by asking the patients to phone in and confirm they needed their delivery, before the delivery date. If the patient forgot to phone in they would have to buy pads until a delivery could be arranged, as each base did not have more than a few pads for emergencies. Matters improved, though disposal of unopened packs not required remained an issue. CAS or nurses could not take them back on infection control grounds, so the patient had to sort it out. I advised them to donate them to charity.

At Grovelands we had a HNE -health nurse for the elderly, (not an elderly health nurse!), who did the proverbial pop in visits, for older people to see if there were any problems, with health, medication or care. I look back on this as my favourite mentoring/ teaching experience of all. My colleague, one of the few remaining State Enrolled Nurses, bravely decided, despite nearing retirement , she wanted to convert her registration to Registered General Nurse, and asked me if I would be her mentor. Being very enthusiastic she got stuck in with the copious assignments and written work. This made more difficult due to her dyslexia, I didn't know if I was coming or going, I likened her to the lady in the film "Driving Miss Daisy" as we skipped from one tangent to the next. Her fortitude and original ideas to help her patients were based on years of nursing. She had a fresh and amusing slant on care, with remarks such as:

"...I've been playing the piano with my dementia patients" and:

"I'm sending Sid to thai chi for his legs". Between us we muddled through, and the prized and deserved qualification was obtained.

Chapter 15. The Great Big Turd

Part of nursing, inextricably linked with ethics is the foundation from which good safe care is given, and that people can expect a nurse to be fair, kind and honest. On my first ward as a student nurse, I had come across an incident that didn't seem right. I heard a commotion behind the curtains and went to help. The SEN was bodily hauling a patient out of the chair, yelling at her to stand up. It was obvious to me the confused frail patient was unable to stand at all. I helped get the lady comfortable and the incident passed. Not sure what to do, and early in my training I did not report it. The incident stuck in my mind, and I vowed to myself I must speak up in defence of a patient if I felt uncomfortable about anything in the future.

The Nursing Code of Conduct, set by The General Nursing Council, (professional governing body) is produced to protect the patient, and equally the nurse in her duties, as a framework of response for a difficult situation. An example of this is disclosure, where a patient is about to divulge something that I must promise not to repeat. Before they proceeded, I would interrupt, to make them aware that I may have to take the matter further, as my code of conduct must be upheld, depended on what they wanted to disclose. If the disclosure had already been made, the patient could become angry, but the code still stood.

An elderly bed bound lady told me at a visit, that a

male carer had touched her inappropriately, she didn't want anyone to get in to trouble, and asked me not to tell the care agency. Knowing her well, and the giggly way she told me, I thought she had probably made it up, but could not be sure, and made it clear to her, that because of what she had told me, I had to report it for her safety. In a case such as this the trust Adult Abuse Policy backed my decision to take the matter further. This policy covered five types of recognised adult abuse: social, financial, physical, sexual, and psychological, and gave clear instruction of how to proceed. The incident reported to the trust adult abuse team, went to social services, and could have involved the police if there had been immediate danger. There was also a requirement in a serious allegation for a senior trust manager to be contacted immediately. On that particular day none of them could be found, a worrying time for me. Social services investigated in the short time frame allowed, and found no evidence of any abuse. A storm in a teacup as I suspected, the patient had no idea how much concern and work she had caused, but as a trained nurse I had reported as my duty of care dictated, and not ignored a comment that might have been true.

Patients and their families have the luxury of ignorance as far as a written ethics code is concerned. This meant they could unknowingly be at odds with professional ethics, in their bid to do the best for their loved one. Pat an Irishman, had arrived on his nephew's doorstep in Waverly Road from America. With fairly advanced dementia, it amazed me he had managed to navigate two international airports, to arrive in Reading on the bus, and find the address. His nephew, married with two young children welcomed him in, with no question that he could not live with the family. In their well meaning and chaotic way, they looked after uncle, who they found had a pronounced urinary incontinence, due to his dementia. He knew he needed to pee, and urinated anywhere he happened to be. His nephew, who worked nights, responded by removing all soft furnishings from downstairs, and locking the door as he worried uncle would get lost if he got out.

Pat used to fall, and after one of his admissions, came home with a urethral catheter to manage his incontinence. The family thought it the best thing since sliced bread, no peeing in the sitting room any more. From a nursing stand point it was disaster. A dementia patient may fiddle with a catheter, and pull it out with the balloon inflated, damaging the urethra. (The ten millilitres of water in the balloon has to be removed before the catheter is withdrawn). Secondly Pat did not understand that the catheter had to be changed at least every three months, he protested loudly, and the catheter change resembled all in wrestling, with his nephew happily holding him down, and Pat shouting: "F--k off f--k off". I discussed the reasons for leaving the catheter out with the family, and they would not hear of it, saying with two young children, they could only continue to look after him if the catheter remained.

Recently Pat had had some respite in a residential home to give the family a rest. He came home with a stage four pressure sore on his heel (the most serious sore down to bone). The sore occurred because he had been sedated, for tapping residence on the head, and stealing their dinner. Consent must be gained for any nursing procedure, otherwise it is counted as assault. Pat made it clear he did not want the catheter changed, and his poor cognition meant he could not comprehend the need for the catheter, for the family to keep him at home. I discussed the situation with my colleagues and his doctor, which was that in Pat's best interest, he needed to remain at home. Then by chance I found a solution to the catheter change problem. At the next catheter change, as the nephew was about to spring into action, on a whim I grabbed an apple from the side board, and gave it to Pat. To my surprise he relaxed, and started chomping away. As long as the procedure could be completed before he finished eating the apple, the problem was solved, with novel distraction therapy.

Further along the road I had a patient with breast cancer and advanced metastatic disease of her bones. She lived with her husband, both teachers, they had looked up everything that they could about June's illness. In consequence they became firm advocates of herbal therapy, and held great belief in a doctor they engaged privately, who specialised in alternative medicine. June said she had lost all faith in western medicine, after radiotherapy and chemotherapy, failed to cure her, and had made matters worse with nausea, sickness and hair loss.

On my assessment visit her reluctance to take any medication, other than a herbal remedy for pain, meant her pain score reached nine out of ten (zero no pain, ten worst pain). With her advanced disease and pain level, adequate morphine would have been beneficial, yet June took only occasional paracetamol, with minimal effect. June believed passionately that her private doctor could stem the flow of disease with alternative treatment, and for this he had requested a central intravenous line to be inserted for administration. I discussed this with June's GP, who referred her for a line at the local hospital.

June had requested the initial visit as she needed help in administration of daily coffee enemas, again from her private doctor. I explained to June I could tell her how to administer her enema, but that I would be unable to participate on ethical grounds, as the effectiveness of the treatment had not been proven under the rigorous trials required for patient safety. My colleague who also visited, reported that the private Doctor had forbade cups of tea, of course June did not allow herself this drink that she loved, and would have been a great comfort to her.

The next time I saw June, the central line had been inserted, and the medication prescribed from her private doctor. My heart sank as I read hydrogen peroxide, and examined the multi dose screw top bottle. Both the type of medication, and the packaging were totally inappropriate for intravenous use. Any medication for intravenous use is in a sealed, sterile, one dose vial, not a normal bottle, and hydrogen peroxide is a well known cleansing agent, for topical use only. June and I discussed that because of my ethical code, I could not participate in this treatment. Her GP felt we had both been duped by June's doctor, and checked he had a current licence to practice. I rang the private doctor up, who became very defensive about his treatment, and the GP took the matter further. All I could do was visit and support June as she struggled with her treatments. Pain, and rapid decrease in strength overtook her, and June agreed to morphine, for a comfortable few days before death.

My code of ethics gave an expectation to patients, of how I behaved towards them. Equally I expected to be treated as one human treats another, in a fair kind and honest way. Most patients are wonderful towards their visiting nurse, and negotiation of visit time, treatment, provision of a hand washing facility and so on, would be reached on an amicable basis to suit both parties.

I inherited a quadriplegic patient, paralysed from neck down, from my predecessor, for care of his supra pubic catheter (inserted into the bladder just above the pubic bone, instead of through the urethra). The first couple of visits he turned on the charm, though surprised me by the way he spoke to his live in carer. He ordered them around like a slave, and had a different carer each visit, and my predecessor had said he put her on edge. Over the months this attitude extended to me, being treated as a complete imbecile was not something I was used to or liked. In my line of work I changed many catheters and had become very skilled in the procedure. With this patient if there was going to be a problem, he had it. Coupled with this he knew best as to how the procedure should be conducted, and told me in no uncertain terms, despite me explaining to him about our guidelines for catheterisation. I did my best to win him round, to no avail, and I started to dread the visit.

For a while I visited with a colleague for moral support. Then things came to a head. On a particularly busy day he phoned to say the catheter leaked, and he wanted to go out. Bending over backwards to accommodate him, he started shouting down the phone. I decided enough was enough, and that I, nor anyone else, should be bullied. The Bullying at Work policy, covered both staff and patients, I discussed this with my manager, and put in a complaint. His GP and a second doctor saw him to discuss his behaviour. Initially things improved, and then he reverted to his old ways. This time as had been explained to him by his GP, he was removed from the surgery list, and his care circulated round neighbouring surgeries every six months. I wished this could have been resolved another way, and I felt for my colleagues who had to see him for care. The fact that I did not need to see him again proved a huge relief to me, and all things considered I was glad I had taken a stand, and not allowed him to go on unhindered in his dreadful treatment of others.

Here I have strayed a little from the ethical theme of this chapter, to incorporate an example of the boundary of responsibility that led to a funny incident, about a subject close to a nurse's heart, bowels. Grovelands surgery covered several small family run Residential Homes, to which one or other of our little team were frequent visitors. To me these homes were slightly dismal places, out dated in both décor and modern facilities, with the sitting room set out, so all the residents sat round the edge with the television on. The owners and the staff did their best to make life good for the people there, but the surroundings did not help. I visited one day to attend to a gentleman with constipation. On examination he had not had his bowels open for a week, and the rectum was loaded with faeces. I gave him suppositories and adjusted his laxative, and left him for nature to take its course. The next day the manager of the home rang up in a flap. She explained the gentleman had passed such a large turd (as the patient aptly named it), that it had completely blocked the lavatory. The plumber had been called to unblock the toilet, and could I do anything about it?. A bit taken aback I put my hand over the receiver, and had a quick consultation with my colleagues. The unanimous decision was no, we couldn't possibly be responsible for the turd once outside the body!

Chapter 16: All Change and Egg on the Ceiling

Shortly after I started community nursing Berkshire HA (Health Authority) and all other HAs in Britain disbanded in favour of PCTs (Primary Care Trusts) that separated hospital from community. Reading, Newbury and Wokingham PCTs covered West Berkshire, I came under Reading PCT. These three trusts became one, West Berkshire Health and Community NHS Trust, then split into Reading and Newbury PCTs. These trusts then changed to West Berkshire NHS Trust, and finally Berkshire NHS Healthcare Foundation Trust, that covered the whole of Berkshire. That amounted to six different employers for me, a new organisation every six years of service. The original health authorities had gone virtually unchanged since Bevan set up the NHS in 1948. New drugs, treatments and equipment available meant that a radical approach to running the organisation had to be made to keep up with cost and patient expectation. Health authorities received money automatically from the government every year, trusts now had to generate their money like a business, and be penalised if certain targets were not met.

Many of the non clinical decisions that affected everyday clinical work came from the government and health minister, who had the unenviable task of modernising the NHS, with finite resources. A ten year vision for improvement, commenced by the

Labour Government in the 1990s "Tony's Plan", led to more funds for hospital upgrading, and a review of nurses wages that had fallen behind the national average. Extra investment, demanded both tight financial control, and all policies and procedures had to be over hauled. The reason for this scrutiny checked that money was not being wasted, and aimed to improve standards within budget, where by lessening the risk of trusts being liable for large compensation claims.

For me and those I worked with, each time the trust reorganised meant changes that affected us. There would be a new logo, so immediately all the documentation would be out of date, boxes of existing stationary thrown out, and all existing care plans in the patient's home re-written. Not until the final county wide change to Berkshire Healthcare NHS Foundation Trust, did managers agree what a waste of money this caused, and previous stationary could be used until it ran out, before starting the new supply.

In line with the new business acumen GP surgeries became fund holders, and employed a practice manager to look after the business side to ensure the surgery achieved income related targets. Grovelands now had to pay for the community nursing service, and in turn charged the trust for the rental of rooms used by community nurses at the surgery. The doctors decided they wanted a CHNE (community health nurse for the elderly), the trust obliged, and this nurse, employed by the trust saw only Grovelands patients. Surgeries could employ directly, one had a chest specialist physiotherapist, and another a community health nurse for the elderly. In future years the employment of these staff worked in their favour, as they kept the service. On the other hand the CHNE at Grovelands employed by the trust, had to cover three surgeries, an equality of services initiative. My manager got very cross when I inferred this was a dilution of service in the name of equality.

The powers that be decreed that DN teams should integrate with health visiting teams. At a large meeting at Bayer's Drug Company Headquarters in Newbury, several of us tried to understand how this would work, as the two jobs were different in those patients seen and health issues treated. Both sides tried to explain this to management. HVs and DNS always had referred to each other. We discussed that if on a visit the HV had a concern about granny, and vice versa if a DN had a child concern, we always referred to our colleagues in the other service, and we were at a loss of how much more we could integrate. Management proceeded anyway, and Self Managed Integrated Nursing Teams, known as SMINTs commenced. Looking back I think this was far more about integrated budget, not nursing, though this was not how it was presented.

When the SMINTs were being set up, everyone from

all teams had to attend team building, so that we could get to know our HV colleagues better, the ones we saw on a daily basis at the surgery. This entailed an afternoon in a school hall at Stoneham Court. The new trust trainer turned out to be obsessed about Reading Canoe Club, we heard a lot about that, and volunteer work on the Kennet and Avon Canal. This immediately got my back up, as voluntary work took overtime from the banksmen, money my husband and his colleagues relied on to make up low earnings into a living wage. We were divided into four teams, and given a pile of sticks, string and paper. My heart sank as the task revealed itself, each team had to get an egg off the ceiling. Yes, on the ceiling four raw eggs had been taped, and the team had to get it down unbroken with the equipment provided. Before entering into the team spirit required, I remember looking round the room at all those trained nurses, and marvelling how money could so easily be saved. I never had been over keen on team building games, and can safely say the egg on the ceiling escapade put me off permanently.

My colleagues and I, after training, could now interview and engage new staff members, previously carried out by our manager. The assumption that the personnel department would do most of the donkey work proved inaccurate. An employment pack arrived in the post, and we did everything else. This included job specification and description, advert, screening applicants, interview, and offering the successful applicant the job, with all the necessary paperwork. We didn't mind this new duty as we decided who to employ, it just took away so much clinical time. After interview certain applicants were easy to discount, one, in answer to a question shrugged her shoulders and said that not much could be done for old people, so she was out.

The pros and cons of other interviewees made our decision more difficult, and then it would not be until they started that we really knew how they worked. The HCA post came up most often, and we had varying success with this. One HCA always put paraffin gauze on a wound regardless of what she didn't read in the careplan, or our clear explanations. Another, in her pronounced northern accent when asked about a wound, always said: "Well, it loooks a bit mucky", no amount of description of what had to be reported changed this declaration. The third developed a phobia of taking blood, a most important and frequent HCA duty. Despite copious training under supervision, and being sent to easy to bleed patients, she would ring to say she had trouble, so one of us had to visit anyway. Thankfully the final HCA employed turned out to be a hard working salt of the earth person, who is still at Grovelands today.

We each had a different admin job in the SMINT, one of the HV's did budget management. On a monthly basis a man came form finance and went through our spend, oddly he could never tell us how much budget we had, and none of us understood how we could run SMINTs without this information. When the HV left, I inherited the job and the petty cash. I had a request for a petty cash balance. I gave finance the figure, nineteen pounds and two pence, and said, as we didn't need petty cash it would be returned. According to finance there was a ten pound discrepancy, I explained the fund had been inherited, and I had no explanation. The amount of time and forms this generated must have cost ten pounds to return the cash.

Soon after the surgery became fund holding the first computer arrived in our office. I looked forward to this, as I was sure it would make life easier. Everyone had tuition, and a password to use Torex and Sophie, the patient record systems. Some surgeries chose to use other systems, unremarkable at the time, this had repercussions fifteen years later. Communication started to join up, and none of the systems in surgeries or hospital would connect with each other. For me in the DN team, access to patient records from our room seemed really novel and saved time, as I no longer had to physically pull files from the carousels in reception. The GPs had a tiny favour to ask, that we put a note on the patient record on their computer, so they also had a record of our nursing care. We explained that written notes were made in the house, and in the hard notes in the office. However it did not take long, and was soon absorbed into the daily routine.

Because of the dynamics of community nursing, the careplan would be left in the house, so any visiting nurse had a record to refer to, and complete for the next visiting nurse. Back in the office, a second set of hard notes were kept, so we had notes to refer to for phone calls, talking to the doctor and so on. So we started to make a third entry on the computerised record. It proved impossible to drop either of our two written records, as legally they belonged to the Trust that employed us, not the surgery who had their own set of records. This annoying duplication continued for years, and has only recently begun to make progress. Everything slowly became computerised; one of the first things to go was our Friday folder, sent out each week with policy updates, training dates and so on. Instead we received individual emails, personalised training reminders, and a host of other information to read and action.

Policy for computer use had to be hastily written after an incident in Caversham. The DN at one base noticed that her student nurse spent an inordinate amount of time on the computer. She assumed this was for study purposes, until she looked over their shoulder one day, to see not nursing research and literature, but adult material of the pornographic variety!

In the early days of computerisation, no one realised how important it would be to have one system for everyone, and the impact programme change would cause. All the nursing teams based in a surgery had a surgery email address. the Trust became computerised slightly later than the surgeries, so staff at head quarters had a trust email address, and then issued all their nursing staff with a second email address. I stayed with the surgery email, as to have two seemed ridiculous. Then it was decreed the surgery email addresses would be discontinued, and all trust staff change to the national NHS.net system. This seemed a good system, with a national global address book, excellent for new networking as it came to be called. As often happened in the organisation, that particular manager left, and the full change over never materialised. A few years on and the trust sent out yet another new email address for all staff. I reminded them of the benefits of NHS.net, and declared I would continue with one email as before, however I did arrange emails to be forwarded from the other account. All new initiatives in my opinion should be fully implemented, followed up, and run for a minimum of two years before change to something else.

Professional Development Plan (PDP) gave a prime example of what I called seagull management. Namely, someone who flew in, made a huge commotion, and sodded off. Cynically I am sure this type of manager had no interest in their current job, other than to prove they could manage change, for their CV, and ladder progression. I attended the training for the Electronic Record System (ERS), with everyone else in the Trust. ERS proved comprehensive and complex, so as my Staff Nurse's PDP fell due, we asked the tutor to talk us through, so we completed it correctly. This she duly did, and announced she would leave for a different department next day. A month later her successor gave all staff a smart folder complete with logo for their professional development. I couldn't believe staff were not only going back to a paper based system, but also all the training and expense of Trust subscription to ERS was for nothing. About ten of us persevered online. Years on the trust stopped the ERS subscription, I moved my PDP into Microsoft Word, the retrograde step to paper, not for me.

Staff grades returned to Bands 123..., to replace existing grades ABC.. In an initiative to include staff for re-banding, G Grades myself included, were invited to a meeting to discuss the new bands, to see how we would slot in. We all had a list of our accomplishments ready; I and others had not forgotten the last grading fiasco. This got twisted round into the more achieved, the more had to be proved. In fact G Grades became Band 6, with a yearly increment as before, and received a pay rise, as did the staff nurses who went from E Grade to Band 5. However not everyone did well. A colleague of mine had been granted an F Grade for outstanding service, in effect a junior sister's post, and unusual in the community. Her F Grade became a Band 5, with protected pay for five years, this meant no pay rise during that time, and a possible drop at the end of five years if the salary had not caught up with her protected pay. Senior health care assistants, given the same band as their hospital counterparts, reluctantly elected to drop advanced skills like doppler and continence follow up. Hospital HCAs at the time worked at a more basic level, yet would be paid the same. How de-motivating and unfair for these staff, and none of us able to do anything about it.

Until policies were updated, many procedures had guidelines instead. A guideline should be followed unless a good reason can be made for straying from it, where as a policy must be followed to the letter. A colleague and I had been asked to update the wound care guidelines, and under wound cleansing wrote "to cleanse or not to cleanse, that is the question" as a sub title. We had a visitation from the DNPG (District Nurse Professional Group), our tone was too flippant, and did we not know the guideline would now become policy, and that there was a policy for writing polices?

My staff nurse reported a patient had been abusive. As it happened I had recently attended risk management training, and the person from the risk department had said he was more than happy to visit a DN team if they had a problem. We met up, explained what happened, and he dictated a stiff letter, that I sent to the patient. A week later I had a call from management who wanted to see me about a complaint, and was hauled over the coals about the letter that had been sent. The text had not followed procedure, or the template letter in the policy. I argued that we had had expert advice from the risk team, who should have known his own policy that he had written. But no, because, as line manager for my staff nurse, I should have read the policy. There were around a hundred and twenty policies, some at least a hundred pages long, ones used regularly I knew well, ones that I seldom used I asked for advice, lesson learnt, read the policy come what may. Clinical policies that set out how when and why, are now paired with Standard Operating Procedures, SOPs, these incorporate a step by step tick sheet in the patient's careplan. Back in my training, on each hospital ward we had a procedures folder, SOPs looked very similar to me albeit under a different guise.

Chapter 17: The Steady Stream of Change

To keep track of change, improvements or efficiencies that had to be made, data collection became more. When I started at Circuit Lane we had a hand held Infalog, once a week this involved a trip to Dellwood where our manager was based, to download information entered in the week. The nurses didn't see any benefit from this, and it became superseded by two different paper versions, and eventually went on line, it would be years until data collection proved useful to nurses. Alongside our working data we went through spates of data collection for other aspects the trust required statistics about.

One of these, for patient satisfaction required us all to submit a monthly return, this involved a list of any gifts received from a patient. Trust policy frowned on gifts, in case it promoted favouritism and put staff in a difficult position. Small gifts of a value less than ten pounds were acceptable. The first Christmas I worked on the community I had the experience of returning a monetary gift. This grand elderly lady had sold up to the developers, her large country house demolished, and retirement homes built on the sizeable plot. She moved into her substantial new build, complete with majestic brown furniture that dwarfed the house, and two large Alsatians who covered the entire place in dog hair. When I opened the card she handed me earlier it contained forty pounds for the children. Over the weekend I agonised over this, as I knew she would be very affronted if I returned the money, and she was, exclaiming it would only go to the taxman.

Anyway, back to the trust data collection to gage patient satisfaction. I had some odd gifts, and felt obliged to list then correctly to prevent data skew. One return read: "old watch, strap broken no mechanism, two chocolate bars three years out of date" and, my favourite "one boiled sweet sucked and carefully re-wrapped". It tempted me to write a million pounds to see if anyone looked at all this information.

There was a steady stream of changes to the everyday equipment, either due to improvement or safety. The yellow multi-use vacutainer holders, used to hold the needle and the vacuumed bottle for venepuncture (taking blood), changed to a white one use only. The green mushroom shape needle receiver went out of use, the used needle now went straight from the patient into the sharps bin, and cut the risk of needle stick injury. Dressing packs came with sterile sheet, apron and gloves, cotton wool and gauze swabs were removed as they were often wasted, and could now be added separately if required. At one time there had been talk of community nurses taking any rubbish created away in their car, the trust were worried about infection control of rubbish. A small amount of dressing rubbish had always been put in the household bin at the patient's house, and a yellow bag collection organised with the council for large amounts. Everyone went up in arms about transporting rubbish in the car, special plastic box or not. None of us wanted rubbish in the vehicle used for the family, and the idea never came to fruition.

The vehicle used for work had to be a comfortable reliable partner, Alistair as a car fanatic loved to change cars, and his interest led to a succession of ownership. When I started community work I had a Montego inherited from my father, plenty of room for kit, but developed an annoying habit of the boot lid popping open over a speed bump. Next I had a Ford Escort estate, roomy and practical for family and work, it over heated and cooked the engine. The automatic Vauxhall Astra replacement had a special button with a snow flake on it, I put great faith in that button sliding down Dee Road one winter, and it never let me down. Having said that I managed to negotiate a slippery Brunswick Hill in my Citroen Pluriel, with no special button, and in summer that car had an electric fold back roof which got rid of the heat on hot days. On short trips between visits the air con' never got going quickly enough in the cars I had. My favourite of all time was the Mini Cooper S, with all the bells and whistles (extra gadgets and chrome). In town driving there was little scope for maximum potential, so to add spice to life I used to set the cruise control and hold thirty miles an hour through clear roundabouts along the Oxford Road.

Charlie and Georgette had both grown up, so no longer in need of a family car we bought an Audi TT sports model. A super car with a good size boot, but otherwise a little impractical for the job, especially in snow. For speed and handling it had fifty fifty weight distribution, and low profile tyres. With insufficient weight over the drive wheels, if I crept forward to start on snow I might get away, usually the spade came out. I love snow, but not at work, where most of the driving would be on uncleared side roads, I resorted to areas that were cleared of snow, or flat so I could park without getting stuck, and walked the rest.

The final car for work wafted me along in air conditioned comfort and black leather seats, complete with reversing camera parking sensors, blue tooth etc. Apart from being a bit of an old man's car, according to Alistair, the Honda CRV gave a sense of luxury and calm to the working day.

While at Grovelands the New Millennium happened. There had been all sorts of rumours that a Millennium Bug, would strike at midnight of the New Year, and disrupt all organisation computers creating havoc, thankfully it proved to be rumour. It was a special time to celebrate a New Millennium, everyone had a party planned. My family met up at Myles and Helen's (brother and sister in law), for a beach party, complete with sand, BBQ and swimming costumes in the house. I had the honour of knowing two patients, who in their early hundreds had not only spanned two

Millennium, but three centuries to boot, what an accolade.

I worked in a happy stable team, and all in our forties we vaguely wondered if we would see retirement out from our present position. Little did we know the trust were about to invoke their powers, and we would have no say in the matter. Originally two district nursing sisters ran each base. Gradually the teams changed as skill mix came in, where, when one sister left, she was replaced by a staff nurse. My colleague came in one day and dropped an unexpected bombshell. Management had decreed she must move permanently to another team in East Reading, to sort out various problems. Whatever we or the GPs said made no difference, trust policy had a clause that staff could be moved if the business need dictated, and that was that. It was the speed and execution of the move that proved particularly upsetting to us, especially my colleague. We three still meet up and reminisce about the great times we had together at Grovelands.

Our team settled down as best it could, and we had a succession of staff in what had been a long term stable post. First, a great DNS recently qualified, whose heart was elsewhere, and transferred as soon as her favoured post became available. Then there were two staff nurses. One left to have a baby. In our team before my colleague was moved, we joked that we could only have members that worked full time, and no pregnancies or sickness, due to the paper work generated. I thought back at this observation, while ploughing through admin caused by these staff. The second, friendly and likeable, proved to be a bit of a loose cannon, and accident prone, car trouble? keys locked in the boot?, guess who. They moved on to a post closer to home.

Years passed, and I began to feel restless, and decided if I were to make a career change, the time had come. I started looking round, and applied for the new tissue viability specialist's post (advising on wound care).A specialist post meant becoming a real expert in one field, at the expense of a broad knowledge of all sorts of conditions as a general nurse. Unsure if I wanted a specialist post I applied for interview practice anyway, and the post went to a colleague of mine who had already set up a Tissue Viability Service elsewhere.

At the start of 2009 the Trust started talking about two new posts that encouraged career progression. These were as a TL (team leader) to run several DN teams, or a CM (community matron) to case manage people with a chronic condition, and reduce admission to hospital. Team leader did not appeal to me at all, as clinical work would be reduced to a minimum. However the community matron post really got my attention, there had been a successful three year pilot study in the trust, and they decided to roll out and formalise the job. Though in effect a specialist post, it incorporated the general aspect I enjoyed. I prepared carefully for that interview, read up on the government papers "The Essence of Care", and the "Seven Pillars of Clinical Governance", updated my CV and off I went. The investment of time and study in my degree, and Independent Nurse Prescribing qualification paid off, and the post was mine.

There were ten new CM posts, and senior staff nurses were encouraged to apply for the vacant sisters posts. Those SNs who were successful did not have the district nursing qualification that those vacating the posts had, so they became CNS (community nursing sisters), instead of DNS. Those of us leaving the post did point out how important this qualification was for the job, and sure enough some found the role really difficult, especially the extra responsibility for staff it entailed. A few years on the trust realised what we had said, and everyone had to complete the DN course as part of their PDP career progression.

In the near future the term district nurse will probably be dropped, an end of an era, in favour of the title Community Nurse Practitioner that might better reflect the new complexities of community nursing. I talked my SN into applying for my post with success, and I knew the team would be in good hands. I said farewell to patients I had known for years. Grovelands staff did a lovely lunch time leaving event for me, with kind words, flowers and gifts, all a bit of a whirl. My work world was about to dramatically change, it felt like jumping off a cliff.

Chapter 18: Camaraderie and Exciting Times

I knew all the matrons and the three team leaders, they had been colleagues for years, and we were about to embark on an exciting career adventure. Both posts had to be developed, and we would be instrumental in this process, shaping the services as they evolved. We matrons had a new manager, who, very keen, supportive and intuitive with the fledgling service, managed to stay long enough to get things going before she moved on. The three matrons who did the pilot study were counted in the ten, and one became the main mentor for us new matrons. This colleague had an excellent overview of what we needed to achieve, and made herself readily available for our many questions and queries.

My new office in Dellwood Unit at Prospect Park Hospital had no windows and took a bit of getting used to, apart from that it was great to be based with three of my CM colleagues. We enthusiastically set about our new work, to begin with training took a large part of time, as we up-skilled on examination, body systems, and medication. In the past I had sat in on GP consultations, and this became a necessary part of my CM training to participate and improve my diagnostic skills. It was a privilege to work with these GPs, and gave an insight into the depth of knowledge, complexity, and decisions required of a doctor. Participation in a surgery was a whole different ball game from observation only, and I benefited a great deal from these sessions. The synonym we were taught to use was "OLDCART", standing for Onset, Location, Duration, Characteristics, Aggravators, Relievers, and Treatments. This gave a set method to gather all the information required for a treatment decision. Diagnosis and treatment is ultimately the responsibility and remit of a doctor. However as a CM I needed to be able to recognise and respond to changes in a patient's condition at an advanced level. There developed a great sense of camaraderie as our group attended courses in Oxford, Slough, Bracknell and Reading, we took turns to drive, and chatted away about our work. We helped each other, learnt and planned.

Doors opened up to us in our new posts. I and my colleagues would be invited, and be expected to attend all sorts of lectures, seminars and workshops. At the level we were now expected to work, many of these events were run by consultants, mainly to keep doctors updated in different specialities. CMs became a welcome addition, as the medics started to comprehend how our collaborative roles helped and supported each other, in the overall goal of good safe patient care.

I could understand how medics earned their money, these consultants and doctors made their speciality understandable, despite the immense complexity, and they purveyed an infinite knowledge of their subjects. The neurological team used "Make Love Slowly Every

Afternoon Preferably Before Lunchtime", to help us understand the process of dementia. It stood for loss of Memory, proceeded by difficulty in Language, deterioration in Speech, unable to recognise their Environment, that lead to loss in Attention span, Perception, then Behavioural changes, and finally Lifeline when life systems shut down to result in death. The respiratory consultant referred to "blue bloaters" and "red puffers" as an aide memoir to the collection of symptoms for different respiratory diseases.

Some of the training in the use of our new ECG and spirometry machines used for our medical assessment came from within our CM group. These CMs had worked in the pilot study, or came from another speciality. To understand interpretation of an ECG reading there was William and Marrow, and Barn Door. Markers PQRST are used on five points of the ECG line, and a normal ECG has a standard pattern. The M (Marrow), and W (William) and Barn Door shapes denoted abnormalities in the tracing of the line, the diagnosis of the former escape me, and Barn Door denoted a myocardial infarction (heart attack) in progress. Spirometry required accurate interpretation of the results to distinguish obstruction, restriction or both in lung function of respiratory disease. It also required a good blowing technique from the patient, often the most difficult part as coordination and breath control were paramount for an accurate result.

Every week we met with our Consultant Physician in Elderly Care. Young and very approachable none of us felt unable to bring up a silly question, as we each discussed a patient treatment dilemma at the meeting. On a monthly basis we met up with the Community Palliative Care Consultant, who would also discuss, and see if necessary patients we had a concern about. There would be no problem about contacting either consultant when needed, or them contacting us, and we all respected and trusted both, as they did us.

In the office at Dellwood we worked alongside the neurological rehabilitation, and occupational therapy teams. Right next door were the new heart failure, cardiac and respiratory teams, and later our new consultant physician for the elderly had a room next door. It proved beneficial for everyone, and I had never had it so good before or after, there is nothing like having an expert in their field readily available. Needless to say this ideal did not last, the offices were needed by Dellwood, and everyone moved out. My matron colleague and I went to Southcote Clinic, where I had originally started working at my first DNS post at Circuit Lane Surgery.

The difference between district nurse and community matron can, simplistically be described as one being more surgical, for want of a better word, and procedure bound, and the other, the matron post, more medically orientated. In earlier days of DN work there was more allowance for a holistic approach. That had gradually been squeezed out, due to higher patient turnover, and emphasis on tasks, as these were easy to measure for performance and cost savings. Measurement of community matron effectiveness, the crux of the job, was to record the number of admissions prevented, or the reduction in the length of hospital stay. This would save the Trust money, as they were charged for each admission and length of stay, by the hospital.

To find patients for the CM caseload needed an entirely different approach from that of the DN caseload, where patients would be referred due to a nursing need, wound, catheter, and end of life care for instance. With the new CM caseloads a proactive search would be made for suitable patients, who suffered complex medical conditions, and had had multiple unplanned hospital admissions because of them. Heart failure, diabetes, and COPD (chronic obstructive pulmonary disease), were typical of the diseases we treated. To find these patients we used RISK, a computer programme that held information on all patients in West Berkshire, and could be screened by surgery, age, and condition, number of hospital admissions and so on. It worked well, and identified those that would most benefit from CM help.

This required in depth assessment of the patient, with the first visit up to two hours, and an hour allowed for each subsequent visit. The patient would be taught to look out for danger signs of deterioration in their condition, what to do, and to contact the CM with any problems before they escalated to an admission. However, this proved more of a challenge to measure than number of wounds dressed, bloods taken, catheters changed as in DN work. Hospital admissions may not have dropped, but would these admissions have gone up more, or risen less with CM input at home?. This was a subjective measurement, and difficult for the bean counters to attach a monetary figure.

My contact with my first patients found on RISK proved nerve racking. In effect I "cold called" them, and when trying to sell anything, in this case my free service, it would be success or failure in the first few minutes of conversation. The patient had no idea they were about to be contacted, or what a Community Matron did. I gave my name, title and quickly added that I worked closely alongside their Doctor at the surgery. This got the foot in the door, and enabled me to explain how I could help them keep as well as possible, and cut down the need for emergency admission, and I could visit for a full health assessment. Most people are interested in their own health, and pleased a professional is able to help. Despite the cold call a patient rarely declined. If the patient agreed to the service, I completed a comprehensive questionnaire about their health that took about an hour. By starting the assessment on the phone I cut down the lengthy visit to come, and had valuable background information.

First assessment visits went something like this. Armed with all the information I needed, a new folder for the patient, and my CM kit I set off. For this job everyone had been issued with medical kit. I found an ideal bag for this in the local tack shop, a grooming kit for a horse. It consisted of a navy free standing oval bag, with pockets round the outside. Ideal for carrying pulse oximeter, urine testing kit, specimen pot, wound swab, venepuncture kit, otoscope, electronic thermometer, tuning fork, neuropathy filaments etc. The space in the middle accommodated the sphygmomanometer, stethoscope, subsequent visit forms, and a comprehensive file of information leaflets. All the kit weighed quite a bit, so I mounted the bag and the scales on a folding camp trolley. The trolley, snaked at high speed, and needed skilled control to stop everything falling off!

John, one of my early and long term patients lived close by my base, which turned out to be handy for us both, as he frequently needed my attention. He came in the top five of my eventual caseload of up to forty patients, who had the most admissions, and required a great deal of backup, I saw him every week at least. The majority of more stable patients, were seen once a week, or every two weeks, and a few "back burner" patients I saw monthly. Everyone had my mobile phone number, and could ring me any time for advice, or where to get advice if I was off duty. This caseload represented the top five percent of people frequently admitted, because their chronic condition got out of control, and accounted for the use of a staggering forty percent of emergency hospital beds. These statistics made it clear why the patients on each CM caseload had been identified via RISK for special help and guidance.

I knocked on John's door and waited, and could hear his partner Eve coming to let me in. We went into the small crowded sitting room, and I made my introductions. With advanced COPD (chronic obstructive pulmonary disease, invariably smoking related), John's shoulders heaved as he fought to breath and get his words out, and he flopped back into his chair after he got up to shake hands. He was thin, barrel chested, and had clubbing and spooning of his fingers, all tell tale signs of prolonged respiratory disease and hypoxia (low oxygen level). When I listened to his chest he had reduced air entry on the left base, a slight wheeze, and no crackles that indicated infection was not currently present.

Detailed physical examination on the first visit gave the all important picture of what signs and symptoms John had, that where part of his chest condition, and gave a benchmark on subsequent examination of any deterioration. John had been advised that on this visit I would examine him top to toe, head, eyes, ears, neck, abdomen, limbs, fingers and toes, nothing of note not already mentioned was found. Previous blood tests showed hyponatremia (low sodium), monitored by his GP, and his records showed medication for epilepsy, and he had not had any recent   fits.

We moved on to his medication. He had three different inhalers for his COPD, seretide and tiotropium inhalers, to prevent and reduce airway closure, and salbutamol/ ventolin to relieve breathlessness and relax the bronchioles, plus a nebuliser for salbutamol. Anti-epileptics, co-codamol or paracetamol for an old back injury (John had been a builder),   ranitidine for a past ulcer that also protected his   stomach from the other tablets, completed the list. I asked John if he knew what his different medications were for, and how often he took them. As often happened John had little idea what he took, or what they were for, his partner Eve dished them out, and prompted him to take inhalers for his chest. Permanently breathless, John automatically reached for his salbutamol inhaler or nebuliser, and had a haphazard approach to his preventative inhalers. Together we wrote out a list of what to take when, he nodded earnestly and said it helped, though in reality he still went for the Ventolin, and remained vague about the other inhalers.

Modern medicine is a wonderful thing, and very complicated. From manufacture, packaging, dose, side effects, interaction with other medicines, prescription, access, storage, and comprehension, there are one hundred and one pitfalls to avoid, before the medication is taken effectively by a patient. For a start all medication has at least two names, a pharmaceutical or generic name, and a brand name, where the manufactures rename the drug to make it their own. Paracetamol is the generic name, and a brand name is Panadol, salbutamol is a generic name, and Ventolin a brand name.

A common mistake, in a patient seen by different on call doctors, and found in John's medication, was a prescription for the same drug in a different preparation. In his case Atrovent inhaler (brand name), and ipratropium nebules for the nebuliser. ipratropium is the generic name for Atrovent. Oh for a joined up patient record instead of separate hospital and community ones, John had no idea they where the same drug and took both, doubling the dose.

Drug companies understandably want patients to use their brand, if the brand name could be replaced by the Companies' name the confusion would be lessened, for instance Boots paracetamol and Aventis paracetamol, or Bayers salbutamol. I think this would reduce confusion considerably. The same respiratory drug can be given by different inhalers, as one patient may find a certain inhaler easier to use than the another. John had an impressive array of inhalers in every variety. I helped him find the one he found easiest to use, and sent the rest back to the chemist.

Bear in mind that John found everyday activities of living a huge struggle, let alone taking on the complexity of his medication. People that have a chronic condition like COPD or heart failure are on a gradual down hill trajectory that can last over fifteen years or so. Entrenched in his illness years, the next exacerbation could be the one John might die from, and at best his recovery would be slightly below his previous level of health. This disease trajectory differs from cancer, where once diagnosed people often deteriorate quickly before they die. They do not have the see-saw effect present in chronic disease that is so unpredictable for patient, nurses and medics to manage.

Over the next weeks months and years I saw John many times. He asked me for oxygen, and I explained to him again, that his oxygen level shown on the pulse oximeter did not warrant bottled oxygen, this placated him until the next consultation. We agreed a course of action, a careplan, of what to do if he became more breathless, had an increase in sputum, or a change in sputum colour. He knew to take his salbutamol, and carry out pursed lip breathing to conserve O2 (oxygen) in the lungs, and to phone me. This was where I had a chance of preventing hospital admission, within the hour I would be with him, check his O2 saturation, prescribe a short course of prednisolone (steroid), and antibiotics if required, and reassure him if there was no medical deterioration in his observations.

The trouble came when in breathless panic he forgot

all about his plan, and relapsed to his default of dialling 999. A couple of times the ambulance crew found the CM folder in the house and called me. This worked well as I could reassure the crew that this breathless panic was normal for John. Despite everything he still got admitted by medics who didn't know him. I immediately contacted the hospital and visited the ward to discuss his situation with the hospital staff, to get him home quickly, not easy. However I feel I did save some admissions, and shorten his hospital stays.

Diabetes is an endocrine disease, divided into type one and type two. In type one there is little or no insulin production and usually happens early in life. Type two comes on later in life, characterised by a gradual loss of insulin production, paired with insulin resistance, when instead of carbohydrate entering into cells for later use, it stays in the blood stream, and a raised glucose (sugar) level will register. Raised glucose in the blood stream will, over time, play havoc and cause retinopathy, neuropathy, and nephropathy (damage to eyes, kidneys, and nervous system). People with diabetes are also more likely to have a heart attack, stroke, hypertension (high blood pressure), or atrial fibrillation. Patients often say they have "mild diabetes". There is no such thing, diabetes is a progressive nasty disease, and the reason that good control of diet exercise and medication is so important.

There were a couple of interesting diabetic patients. Evelyn, a genuine type one brittle diabetic had suffered with sudden swings in her blood glucose most of her life. Her glucometer would give a reading of 2mmol per litre, any reading below 4mmol is hypoglycaemia (low blood glucose), and can quickly lead to unconsciousness. Evelyn would have the statutory glucose and follow up sandwich, only to find her glucose registered hyperglycaemia (high glucose), at over 30mmol, fifteen minutes later. Or she would have hyperglycaemia with ketones, where the body, in the absence of carbohydrate for energy, tries to convert fat and eventually protein instead, to then suffer a hypoglycaemic attack shortly after. Along with the diabetes nurse specialist and doctor, we tried all sorts of insulin, diet, and other ideas, to no avail. Of course each time Evelyn ended up in hospital, her insulin would be reviewed and changed, despite liaison with the hospital that this would make no difference to her control, and mean she had to again get used to a different regime. Eventually Evelyn moved away to be nearer her daughter, as Evelyn had had fewer hospital admissions when her husband, who had died, had been able to help her with her unstable glucose.

The other lady, who lived alone, tried hard to adhere to a healthy diet, exercise as much as she could, and take her diabetes medication as prescribed, yet the blood glucose she recorded at various times of the day remained in the teens, (a normal glucose is between 4-7 mmol, with up to 10 mmol acceptable). I had a job to convince the doctor to consider insulin, the next step if oral hypoglycaemics are not effective, due to her long term HBAIC that conflicted with her home glucose results. The blood glucose, taken by a finger prick test will show the level at that moment, the HBAIC blood test shows the average glucose over the previous six weeks. Despite her high home monitoring results, her HBAIC test read within normal range. After discussion with the diabetes nurse specialist, we took a fructoseamine, an alternative to the HBAIC, and sure enough it was well above normal. She started insulin, and the glucose levels settled down. I asked about the anomalies of this at a diabetes conference, and no one could ever explain why the HBAIC result showed normal.

On the whole patients would be kept on once admitted to my caseload, though there where two, who for different reasons were discharged. The first was a lady in her thirties with Graves' disease. Graves' disease is an autoimmune condition of unknown origin that affects the function of the thyroid gland, and can disturb other systems. In this severe case the patient took twenty one different medications, once to four times a day, plus topical skin treatments. The list of consultant care included endocrinology, cardiology, nephrology, dermatology, gastrology, eating disorders, psychiatry, diabetology, and ophthalmology. She was very organised and kept a diary of her appointments, and a file with all her consultant information. Her complex drug regime meant any changes had to be carefully discussed, and usually one consultant needed to refer to another. I could not think of any other way I could help, and discharged her.

The other patient who lived in a run down council house was well known to both health and social care. She was very manipulative of both services, and never showed any intention of taking ownership of her own health. After an admission to hospital she proudly told me she had complained about the cleanliness of her room. I was speechless as I sat in the filthy cluttered kitchen, the new cooker provided by social services ruined, and dog mess on the floor. In a change round of caseload my CM colleague also visited her, a fresh pair of eyes is a great help in this type of situation. Like me, no inclination was found in the patient to help herself, and we both felt our services were more effective elsewhere.

As I said, the majority of patients loved the CM service, but not all. I had a couple of patients that after a few visits did not want to see me again, and other CMs found the same. The first of mine was a morbidly obese lady, whose family were all diabetic and had multiple health problems. When I started to discuss the appalling diet, I tried to think of a small change that could easily be made, and suggested their high sugar orange drinks, could be replaced with plain water. The next time I saw her, she said that this suggestion had upset them all, and could I stop the visits. Lying in state on the sofa, with an enormous body that ended in two dainty feet placed neatly together, a colleague described her as mermaid like, the person listening said she looked more like a slug, an appt description.

It had taken a great deal of explanation to sell my service for this particular patient to reluctantly agree to an assessment visit. I think he only agreed because curiosity got the better of him. When I got to his house I was on best behaviour, and cordially greeted him and his wife at the front door. Unfortunately as I struggled up the steps and into the hall with my kit, I inadvertently clobbered the skirting board. I apologised profusely, and thought they were going to claim against the trust for miniscule paint loss there and then with the fuss they made. Soon after we sat down in the sitting room, his wife asked very pointedly if I wanted to wash my hands. I said it was very kind of them to offer, and dutifully went to wash them, instead of waiting to just before the physical examination, when I washed them again.

The other point they wanted to take me up on was the matter of resuscitation. This has always been a difficult issue to broach, and had supposedly been made easier as it was now included in the assessment. I would bring the subject up as part of my initial phone call. Usually this worked quite well, as if the person did not have a clear view, it gave them time to think about it before my first visit. Some patients brought the subject up themselves and stated clearly they did or did not want to be resuscitated. Others were glad that they were given the opportunity to talk about it, and the occasional patient got offended. My gentleman felt I had already written him off. I explained again that I was obliged to ask all patients if they wanted to be resuscitated, by which I meant after a total collapse, when the heart stopped. The other important part of the information that a patient needed to make an informed decision, was that if resuscitation were to be successful, they may not regain the level of health they had before the collapse. Once the patient had made a decision that they did not want resuscitation they had to be provided with the appropriate paper work known as the purple form, completed by their GP.

Subsequent visits were no easier, despite a health plan to catch his anaemia early that worked well. One day I drew up on the drive, and remembered I had a specimen I had to drop off to catch the morning collection, and pulled out again. Unfortunately I had been spotted on my manoeuvre, and a full scale interrogation took place, as to why I had come and gone when I returned ten minutes later. The final straw was the prickly one of lifestyle changes, and they phoned to say they did not want my input anymore. I breathed a sigh of relief.

Chapter 19: The Job of Community Matron

When I started as a CM I covered two surgeries, Grovelands and Potteries (Tilehurst surgery). Then we changed to work geographically. This meant I saw all patients in one area, regardless of their surgery. The geographic area changed shape, and finally back to surgery patients who belonged to Potteries, Circuit Lane Surgery and Western Elms Surgery. (Commissioning had started, and Grovelands came under a different group). Because of the dynamics of seeing patients in the community, there always had been a dilemma as to whether patients based by surgery or geographical area worked best. Both had their different merits. If I saw surgery based patients the surgeries were in easy reach, though the patients might be more spread out. Especially when I was a DN, it sometimes happened that two nurses visited patients in the same building, who belonged to different surgeries, when it would be more cost effective for one nurse to see both patients. A geographic area meant one nurse could see patients that lived in the same building or road regardless of surgery. However the down side of this, was the patient could be registered with a surgery the other side of town, and this made it more difficult for the nurse to access the doctor if required for that patient. Personally I preferred surgery based nursing, as I not only had good GP access, I got to know them properly as well.

Sometimes we CMs elected to keep a patient on, instead of handing them over when we changed from surgery to geographical working. I had known Sheila for years and decided to keep her on. We had had a good working relationship, she used to call me and say: "Hello mate...", or ring my work mobile answer phone at two in the morning to tell me how she got on at her gardening for dementia, I felt another new face would add to her confusion. Medication and Sheila did not go well together, complete chaos described stock control of her medicines, and how Sheila took her medication from her NOMAD (daily doses made up by pharmacy in sealed trays). At one stage I found she had twenty of all her inhalers and nebuliser nebules, and ten old NOMADs where changes had been made and they became obsolete. To tackle this I phoned both the surgery and the pharmacy who delivered her medication, on a weekly basis, and even then Sheila still had the odd uncalled for delivery.

Around Christmas in the first year of my CM job everyone was affected by the weather. Community nurses are used to working in bad weather, and it took extreme conditions to impact on the service. While at Grovelands we had the heaviest freak rain storm I had ever seen. Each time I got out of the car I got a cold shower, the bungalows on the Bath Road opposite Southcote flooded, so did some houses up on the high ground in Tilehurst. The road drains were so over whelmed with rain water, it came up like a spring from each one, bizarre, and disrupted all the traffic.

That particular afternoon before Christmas I worked at my desk as the sky progressively darkened with snow forecast. It looked so threatening I decided to make for home. As I drove over the railway bridge towards the house there were no cars, and it magically started to snow. I had been home for ten minutes, and total havoc ensued outside on Burghfield Bridge, as cars slipped in all directions. An hour later the whole of Reading became totally gridlocked, a friend of ours took four hours to get to my house from Theale, about three miles away. It happened that Alistair had called in at her house to see her husband, so they swapped suppers and Dave's wife and my husband got to their respective homes several hours later.

The next day I decided I wouldn't take the car, I still had the TT, and being totally useless in the snow, best it remained on the drive. Alistair who had a four wheel drive pickup for work, phoned his boss at CRT (Canal and River Trust), and announced he would offer: "Cross business support for Community Nurses", his boss could not very well say no to this. I down sized my kit into a backpack, put on my wellingtons and off we set. He dropped me at my first patient, then I either walked to the next or he picked me up. One day I walked from Coley Park right up into Tilehurst. The thick snow everywhere looked wonderful, and I was so thankful I did not have to drive. For those without a chauffeur driven service, the Trust had a very sensible approach to work, patients were visited within walking distance of the nurse's house, regardless of surgery. This was particularly apt for staff who had to travel any distance for work. I managed to see all my patients, and so did most other staff.

The snow sparkled in the sun as I crunched towards Cyril's small wrought iron gate, impossible to open with a foot of snow either side. I climbed over and walked up the pristine path, calling out as I let myself in, greeted with: "Hello darling, I didn't expect you today". We chatted about the snow, and a keen animal lover as usual he asked after my dog and pony. Cyril, a tall big heavy man, lived as a widower in his small sparse flat that he wanted to leave to the cat's home. He had all sorts of naval stories to tell, and was fiercely independent. Heart failure and type two insulin dependent diabetes had not been kind to this man, and in the beginning it had been difficult for him to admit he found his extensive medication hard to manage. Like Sheila he could have started a chemist shop with the boxes and boxes of medication he had over ordered. Prone to falls, and extreme breathlessness on walking Cyril still managed to catch the bus up Norcot Hill, to shop in Tilehurst. More often than not he would be brought home by the ambulance crew, called out by a concerned member of the public, when he came close to collapse at the bus stop or in a shop. We used to joke he had taken his personal taxi, i.e. the ambulance to get home.

That morning he had crackle sounds on his chest, and his ulcerated legs were more oedematous (swollen), necessitating an increase of his diuretic (water) tablet for a few days. This turned out to be the one tablet he had run out of, so I wrote a prescription and walked to the nearest chemist to get it for him. I only collected medication like this in emergency, as Cyril had no family.

His health deteriorated and falls increased, with admission to hospital on several occasions. Cyril did everything he could to stay home, and spent a lot of money installing a phone jack point for his patient alarm, and a metal wheelchair ramp to the front door, that cost three thousand pounds. I arranged maximum homecare, but Cyril often declined their help, especially if they were foreign. Despite many discussions we had about this, he would not be persuaded to accept their help. Regrettably he got to the stage that he could not manage between care visits, and he had no alternative but to move to a nursing home. I felt guilty when he finally agreed, because he had tried so hard, and the flat proceeds went on nursing home fees, with nothing left for his beloved cat's home.

Cyril settled into the nursing home and I dropped my visits down to every six weeks or so. Part of the deal he made with me had been, that if he agreed to NH care, I continued to see him. To begin with he hated it there, and determined to get home hatched all sorts of wild schemes, and I would gently reminded him why he went to the NH. Pleased to see me, he did not appear to miss me between visits, so eventually I discharged him. His heart failure and diabetes had stabilised under the twenty four hour care of the home, but I knew where he would prefer to be.

There where some patients who took charge of their chronic condition, and benefited from the extra input I gave, they could work to their careplan, manage their medicines, and recognised a change in symptoms that needed action. I could safely leave them with a short course of steroids and antibiotics in the case of COPD patients, and diuretics in heart failure patients, for them to start and let me know. I then visited, checked them over, gave then a prescription for new emergency medicines, and arranged to visit again as required. In heart failure I arranged a urea and electrolyte blood test. In these patients a careful balancing act required enough diuretic to remove fluid from lungs, limbs etc, without derangement of kidney function ascertained by blood levels. On the other hand I had a couple of patients that I stopped emergency meds for, as they just took them despite the carefully agreed plan of when the meds were appropriate. When I started nursing patients were expected and encouraged to be dependent on nurses and doctors, instead of doing things for themselves.

The upshot of this meant some older patients in particular never did get the hang of ownership of their own health.

Nita, a heart failure of patient of mine in Tilehurst did her best to keep well. She had a pronounced sensitivity to any change in medication, if there was an interaction to have, she would have it, so the GP and I had to be very careful. I would know immediately if she had reacted badly, Nita phoned me and proceeded to report how awful she felt, so I visited to reassess, and often reverted to the previous regime. Not as effective, but at least it didn't upset her. Once I had gone through my health check, looked at her medicines, and made any changes, Nita liked to fill me in on her week. Though her sight was poor, she knitted endlessly for the tiny babies in the Special Care Unit at the Royal Berks, without dropping a stitch, which I found pretty impressive. One day her glasses broke, so she got her son to take her to the opticians. He waited in the car, and Nita went in. She asked the assistant if he could replace the small screw she had with her, and after a tiny pause he said:

"Yes Madam", and disappeared into the back of the shop. Nita sat and waited, and he soon came back with the repaired glasses. He asked Nita where she thought she was, thinking it an odd question she told him. He replied:

" No Madam, the opticians is next door, this is the undertakers!" Nita was barely able to get the story out she laughed so much as she told me, and said everyone had been in stitches when she recounted the incident at Bingo Club.

Several of my patients had warfarin therapy long term for atrial fibrillation, to stop coagulation of blood clots in the heart. This could be fatal if a clot moved in the blood stream, and caused pulmonary embolus in the lungs, or cerebral embolus in the brain leading to a cerebral vascular accident (stroke). Warfarin, a very effective anticoagulant, reduced the risk of a fatal clot forming in the heart had to be regularly monitored with a warfarin blood test, and the dose of warfarin changed according to the clotting time. A normal clotting time of a minute, would be extended up to around two minutes, so the blood would be too thin for a clot to form. If the test showed the clotting time had increased too much warfarin dose decreased to avoid prolonged bleeding, and vice versa. The anti coagulation clinic would then instruct the patient to alter the warfarin dose up or down by adjustment of their brown, blue and pink tablets. Instructions might be:

"Take one pink and one brown, total six milligrams", and after the next test:

"Take one blue and one brown tablet total four milligrams", if the clotting time had risen.

Warfarin is the most effective anticoagulant, though in some patients the risk of over or under coagulation out weighed the benefits. Over the years I had several people that, after discussion with their GP warfarin would be stopped, in favour of aspirin, a less affective anticoagulant that did not require regular blood tests. These patients were unable to alter their dose, as they didn't open the letter with new dose instructions, carried on with the previous dose, or didn't ask the nurse to visit for the next blood test. If their medication came in a NOMAD this presented another problem, if the dose changed often, may be every week, by the time the script had reached the pharmacy and the new NOMAD delivered it would already be out of date. I have known patients to have a clotting time of ten minutes, this put them at huge risk of haemorrhage if they fell and cut themselves or banged their head.

On a visit to one lady who had become way out of control with her warfarin, and had not been coping in general, I entered the house to be immediately confronted by her three very concerned daughters. I explained what care, both health and social would, or would not be available for their mother. The conversation became interspersed with:

"Something must be done" by one or other of the daughters, with hands on hips, as I reiterated what I had said, and this continued for about half an hour. I felt completely frazzled. When a crisis point like this is reached in regard to care, it is not unknown for a family to have expectations way above services that are actually available. I contacted the anti coagulation clinic and the doctor to sort out the warfarin dose and blood tests, and left the family with contact numbers for social services and other appropriate avenues of voluntary help. Back at the office I fed back the visit to my colleagues, and forever after, as soon as one of us put hands on hips, we knew:

"Something must be done!"

My colleague went to great lengths with one of her men, she would take the blood, phone the laboratory for the new dose and next test date. Then go round next morning to change his dose, go and get the new NOMAD from pharmacy, and deliver it back to the man, for his carers to give. Very time consuming. Thank goodness newly developed anticoagulants like rivaroxaban are less likely to cause serious bleeding, stay at a constant dose, and do not need regular blood tests.

I looked after Joan, on warfarin for repeat pulmonary embolus in her lungs, with severe COPD. Joan had her family at home to help her with her warfarin, and everything else. She used to be horrible to them, and yell: "Get in here now...", and they all moved out and left her to carers. She had been a carer herself, and bossed the carers that came to her, nothing was right. As a CM, or if the doctor visited the demands continued, albeit with a better manor. Despite oxygen therapy and maximum respiratory medications her extreme breathlessness made her panic, and fall. Apart from reiteration of routine controlled breathing exercises, nothing more could be done. The change from complicated warfarin to straight forward Rivaroxaban at least kept her safer from haemorrhage.

Joan ended up with multiple emergency admissions. I would even arrange a night sitter after discharge from hospital in an effort to keep her home, but the admissions continued. It is difficult for a visiting on call doctor, or paramedic to have the assurance not to admit a breathless frightened patient they don't know. Despite a specific emergency plan in the CM folder, with a range of base line observations to compare with their own, and what helped in an exacerbation for Joan, the decision to leave a patient at home would be their responsibility, a difficult one. Sometimes despite all my efforts they did not see the emergency plan in the bright yellow folder, occasionally Joan would be stabilised, and I would be phoned for immediate follow up. This was what should happen, and hopefully professionals will start to do this more, instead of taking the easy option to admit the patient. Inevitably the nursing home beckoned, Joan continued to lambaste the carers there, not an easy lady.

Chapter 20: Date Collection by Helmet Cam?

I noticed a steady and increasing trust governance as time past in my CM job. There were two reasons for this, firstly that the organisation strove to improve the service provided, and secondly wanted to provide evidence that improvement had been achieved. I had my own viewpoints as a clinician. I remained fully supportive of the trust to improve and give an excellent health service to patients. The proof of this activity however was more problematical for me. The only way to collect the information for the trust, meant the work force who saw patients, had to record all activity carried out, clinical and non clinical. This had always been required to some degree, but became almost more important than the job of seeing patients. All those teams of people in the trust office, were to a large extent depended on the information fed from the work force to be able to do their own job. To the work force with a priority to see and treat patients, data collection was secondary.

I would ponder data collection, and try to think of a way it could be accurately collected without those who visited patients, actively doing the collection. Everyone I knew tended to use certain codes, when there might be a code forgotten about, that would more accurately reflect the activity recorded. Fairly soon after I started as a CM we had a new data collection program called RIO, which incorporated an electronic patient record element. At least this was a step forward in the reduction of written records. The programme had been written primarily for data collection, and the patient record side seemed a bit of an after thought. Both parts of RIO were complex, this made it easy to miss sections used by some altogether. The data side was not able to pull information out of the patient notes entry made by the nurse. For example if the nurse wrote a blood test had been taken in the patient record, it also had to be recorded by code on the data side. We needed a system that could extract data directly from a patient record, I wonder if this will ever happen?

My tongue in cheek idea was that everyone should be issued with a helmet cam. Confidentiality would be an immediate issue, but with careful thought I am sure this could be overcome, for both patient and nurse. Nurses must be able to take a comfort break without it being recorded. It might take a bit of getting used to, but in the long run solve data collection problems, and in an age of increased litigation, could provide proof of an incident superior to a written document. How the data could be extrapolated is another matter. It may be possible to down load on to a computer data system. However the data, sifted through manually by my proposed new Head Cam Data Collection Team, might raise a few eyebrows when they saw the procedures, crevices, bottoms and folds that are second nature to a trained nurse!

With pressure ulcer monitoring for data collection the

trust, under government dictate, developed a process that could have benefited with one of my suggested collection methods. Pressure ulcers (bedsores), are caused by pressure, friction, or shearing force, preventable in the majority of patients. These came under the spot light as a relatively easy area to monitor for care improvement, with a shift and emphasis on prevention. Pressure ulcers, or lack of them are historically linked with good nursing, and all trained nurses are taught prevention and treatment, and would be mortified if a patient developed a sore under their care. If a patient was very poorly, or near death, their skin might break down occasionally, despite all efforts, and as long as everything had been done, nurses knew they had done their best.

Pressure sores, staged one to four denoted the severity of skin damage. Stage one, a pink non blanching spot, two superficial skin loss, three damage through to the adipose tissue (fat layer), and four damage that involved muscle and bone. A pressure ulcer generally formed over a bony prominence, where little flesh between skin and bone presented a risk area. Sacrum, heel, elbow, hip, and ears, back of head and shoulder blade all needed to be regularly checked. Part of the first visit involved a skin check, and at each subsequent visit. To calculate the risk of pressure sore development Waterlow score would be used. Waterlow, invented by Judith Waterlow, who I had the pleasure of meeting, gave a quick and easy points system on age, mobility, contributing illness and so on. This score denoted if the person fell into low medium or high risk of pressure ulcer development.

If the risk was low the patient received information about skin care, and monitoring. Medium risk patients also received a foam cushion and mattress, and high risk a Pegasus bi-wave alternating pressure air mattress or similar. All had to be documented in the patient record. If a sore stage two or above had been found on skin inspection it had to be reported, and, counted as a serious untoward event and at stage three onwards would be investigated. For nurses this became critical, and showed up any gaps in care, and if negligence had occurred. The in depth online form asked about immediate action, equipment in place, advice previously given to the patient and so on. Who ever reported the sore then had to meet with a member of the tissue viability team, risk team, their manager, and other nurses involved in the care.

These meetings analysed whether everything possible had been done and recorded to prevent a sore, and if not why not? The manager that called these meetings seemed to relish putting staff on the spot, and nobody enjoyed them. Especially when it was trivial, a colleague knew she had given the advisory leaflet to a patient, hadn't actually recorded this, and later found the leaflet thrown under the bed. A lesson in: "If it's not recorded it hasn't been done", even when you knew it had. As I have said before I am all for improvement, and the incidents of stage three and four sores did drop, and emphasis on proof of initial prevention became paramount. It was the punitive and un-collaborative way carried out that no one liked.

Of course it would not be just down to the nurse to prevent sores, a wider team that included the equipment service, carers, pharmacists, medics, physio, occupational therapy, rapid response team, and other specialists who all played a valuable role. For preventative work the supply of equipment had a huge overhaul. When I started as a DNS the stock in medical loans was limited to a ripple mattress, a few cushions, and about two hospital beds, and took at least a week to come, if in stock. Some DN teams fund raised to buy their own equipment to keep at their base, so they could respond quickly. I felt the problem with this was it should not be necessary, as to do the job adequate equipment should be provided by the employer. There would also be the matter of adequate storage and cleaning. In the end the trust called an equipment amnesty, and all equipment was handed in to medical loans so the stock and circulation increased.

After this things continued to improve once the lack of equipment, highlighted by serious untoward investigation, showed up as a primary reason for sore development. In the recent time of commissioning, medical loans, taken over and run by NRS Berkshire

Healthcare Equipment Services made a massive improvement to the loans service. The trust invested millions in equipment for nurses to be effective and safe, the loans store could now deliver equipment on the day ordered, and provide an emergency evening service throughout Berkshire. The loans company were penalised if they couldn't deliver the equipment on time. Collection of equipment no longer required by the patient however, was not as good as delivery, as a robust tracking method for it has yet to be developed.

Myself and the other CMs were sometimes asked to investigate other incidence and complaints. This took time away from clinical work, I added the hours up of one of mine, and discussed with my manager, it had taken two working days in total . The incident involved a patient who had been missed on the DN visit list, and developed a wound infection. To ascertain where communication had broken down I travelled to two different bases, Newbury Community Hospital, interviewed five members of staff, and presented the report to my manager by a tight deadline. My clinical work, the primary call on my time had to take a back burner, as the trust did not have a dedicated person purely for investigative work.

Other fledgling specialist teams sprang up, and developed into a team of four to five nurses. Specialist heart failure, cardiac, respiratory, tissue viability, falls, and infection control were all available for advice. Our Macmillan nurses, taken over by The Sue Ryder Charity Trust became specialist end of life and symptom control nurses, not an easily memorable title. So much advice became available I sometimes felt that I did the job of several other people, as the new teams were too small to do more than an initial assessment visit. Over the years the amount and depth of clinical research had grown out of all proportion, this made being a general nurse impossible without specialist advice, and these new teams became indispensable.

The CAS (continence advisory service) for which I had taught on their digital rectal course for years, had all their sessions taken over by the training department shortly before I left. The nurses in CAS had their training down to a fine art, and they, like me would be very interested to see how the training department could improve on this.

Inevitably the number and intensity of meetings increased, as all the new services valiantly strove to keep up with the demands of each other, and the trust, dictated from the Department of Health. The individual ideas and requests from management, and specialist teams, would be presented as a quick simple task that took no time at all. A mission statement was circulated, the title sounded as though it had come from Star Trek, but was in fact the overall aim for excellent delivery of health care by the trust. Soon after a community vision for the future initiative started. Seconded managers held meeting after meeting, and, it seemed to me continued the Star Trek theme; they came up with a diagrammatic poster with "health silos" dotted around the region. This poster had been produced at an afternoon workshop with a professional artist, at least the play school colours brightened up each base. To accompany the launch there was a "strap line" that we all had to remember and the content of which has escaped me. It was something catchy like the one used by The Three Musketeers: "All for one and one for all". These little tasks added up and collectively became hours, often with a deadline.

For CMs our meetings schedule included daily, weekly, monthly, and quarterly dates for the diary. Each CM met with their DN team daily as we re-integrated in an advisory capacity. We discussed patients, and devised a careplan if required, to enable nurses to adjust treatment and prevent admission. Every week I attended one of my three surgeries practice meetings, on a rotation basis as three a week was too many. A practice meeting of about an hour, attended by GPs, practice nurse, health visitor, DN gave me an excellent place to liaise with that part of the MDT (multi disciplinary team), to discuss patient care.

In addition to the weekly surgery meeting, each surgery had a monthly MDT teleconference to discuss patients identified by the CC (case coordinator). This new post at Band 5 meant searching out patients frequently admitted as an emergency. Most of these had already been identified by the CMs, and the GPs, who had been told by commissioning that they had to participate, gave the poor CC a hard time. Teleconferencing, new to everyone took some getting used to. All those taking part would be given a code by the case coordinator prior to the meeting, and then at the appointed time we rang to sign in. This could be done from anywhere, such as the car, and we did not have to physically go to the surgery. An electronic voice announced that: "Vivien Ogden Community Matron has joined" and the CC would welcome each member, and included colleagues from social services. The system should have had a visual link, unfortunately from day one this never worked. In consequence there would be a long silence, then everyone tried to speak at once, because we couldn't see one another. Meanwhile the CC fought to chair and keep control. Each patient on the list had their care and treatment reviewed, and revised if necessary. It came as no surprise that after about five months, the CC had had enough and moved on.

My favourite meeting, was our monthly Bite Size run exclusively for and by CMs. We met at the Health and Social Services Centre in Whitley, the most central location for everyone, dug out our tea earn and set to. We took it in turns to arrange the afternoon, and might include an outside speaker, updates, a trust manager , short training session to name but a few items on our agenda. The room would buzz with ideas, plans and resolutions as we all caught up with matron news in Reading and Wokingham. Bite Size had originally been set up by our CM mentor to break down all the new information and training we needed, into manageable chunks, hence the name Bite Size.

CMs attended the monthly local DN rendezvous, where our team leader passed on trust information, and fed comments back to management. Then every quarter team leaders DNSs and CMs met at Whitley for what was known as the DN big meeting. It needed a strong chair to keep control of so many attendees, some of whom were extremely vocal, and the meetings could easily overrun with fruitless banter. The meetings were a larger version of the monthly meetings, and senior managers such as our community nurse manager, and head of adult services manager attended.

For me the most onerous of meetings were the ones arranged by management, at trust head quarters on the Bath Road. They usually included the next long winded and complicated way to collect a vital piece of data, by tomorrow, or how community services could cover more hours with existing resources .QOF (quality and outcome framework), and CQUIN (commissioning for quality and 1nnovation) became all consuming, with one manager or another on the phone, desperate for the next vital data deadline. Our

NM tried her best to lighten the pressure, and referred to CQUINS as pretty sparkly Sequins, and this did raise a few smiles.

The GP surgeries came under the same scrutiny from those commissioning their service, and a couple of the surgery partnerships dissolved a few years later, the management side taken over by the trust. GP practices are in effect a separate business, and those GPs in the ones that would be taken over, made the brave decision to dissolve the partnership of many years. They felt they were no longer able to concentrate adequately on their clinical work, because of the constant call for them to attend to QOF, CQUINS and CQCs (care quality commission). Some of the GPs left their surgeries to work on Westcall, the out of hours doctors service. As one of them said to me, he could see his patients for the whole shift, treat them, write up the notes and go home, with no interference to his clinical work.

The move toward twenty four hour cover from the Department of Health, led to an already fully stretched service extending cover. My Monday to Friday job would soon include Saturday am, and late shifts on a rota basis. There would be no one to cover my patients, who were used to being able to phone me any time in core working week hours, while I had my time back. The whole point of my preventative job seemed to be at risk to a tide of reactionary response. The changes dictated were then down to us to decide how to implement , come what may.

Occasionally we could use the data to our advantage, to push for something CMs required, and obtain a small victory At our nursing conference I enjoyed the enthusiasm from the different nursing and other departments in the trust, as they presented their achievements in the past year. This rekindled the spark of camaraderie, and the drive to give a good safe service to patients, everyone's common goal. I had my own victory here, and came away with a great sense of satisfaction. Along with other senior managers, Helen Director of Nursing for the trust attended. For months I had tried to get a definitive answer about a record keeping issue.

For each patient seen by a CM, we filled out a carbon copy form to record the content of the visit. One copy would be left with the patient. The other we took back to base, and scanned onto the patient record. To start with I shredded the paper copy once scanned, until someone got cold feet, and decreed that they all had to be kept, so much for paperless. I tried several times to get this issue resolved, and no one would make a decision. Here was my chance, straight to the top. I explained to Helen what was going on, and how ridiculous it was, to keep a paper record that had been uploaded onto the electronic patient record, by me using my password. A few days later I received an email that I carefully kept, from Helen that confirmed paper records could be shredded.

Due to the accumulation of calls that took time away

from the job of seeing patients, the government issued an initiative called Compassion in Practice, this incorporated the six Cs, care, compassion, competence, commitment, communication and courage. It had become necessary to remind some nurses about the very essence of their job, and I am sure this would not have been required if nurses had less non clinical calls on our time. The Essence of Care was a further initiative from the Department of Health (DoH) that provided a framework so trusts could prove patients received good care. It had been aimed at hospital care, and statements such as "every patient must be offered three nutritious meals a day", were impossible to implement with people in their own homes.

Every base had to keep a large Essence of Care folder of evidence, made up by one person so the folders were all the same, and the Trust could tick the box for the DoH that evidence had been provided. For some reason a paper version was insisted on, not an online version that would have been easy to access and review. No one ever looked at the folder unless it had to be updated. However we were all expected to know what was in the folder, in case we had an inspection from the CQC, as the trust strove to obtain top marks in care to achieve their payment targets. Both the six Cs and Essence of Care in themselves were long and wordy, took time to implement and it could be said these initiatives compounded the very problem they tried to solve, as nurses time would be taken from direct patient care.

In my early days I knew most of the management based at headquarters at Bath Road, this changed as the trust fluctuated and grew in both size and scope of responsibility demanded by commissioning. For the business of commissioning, the Trust split into two, care provision, and care purchasing, this fuelled the burgeoning management structure. Now it seemed, managers came and went like a dose of salts, as they were seconded, moved on, side tracked or just disappeared. The chief pharmacist disappeared, she had been very vociferous in her emails to doctors and nurses, and decreed what dressings and medicines could be used when. One day the emails stopped, and no-one ever heard from her again. At least our community nurse manager stayed constant, and on the whole cheerful, despite the unenviable pressure from management above, and nurses below.

Chapter 21: Freedom!

Alistair and I, like most couples had thought about what it would be like not to work, with:

"Wouldn't it be great if we didn't have to work", and:

"If we won the lottery..." Once we both turned fifty the idle conversations turned to:

"If we retire..." Retirement seemed a strange and fascinating combination of freedom, and poverty where we would both have more time, with less money to spend. I found myself sifting through the contents of the house, and several items succumbed to eBay and Freecycle, as, if we were to move on in the future, I would not want to take them. For both of us the constant pressure at work began to take its toll.

One Sunday evening I suddenly found myself with a dread of going to work next day. This had never happened before, and I didn't like it. I felt I had had a glimpse of depression. I had always remained firm about my work life balance, and been careful not to let my personal life affect me at work, and tried never to take work home, I worked full time, and had a full time home life. As a fit healthy individual I had only had ten days off sick in my working life, which included a minor operation under anaesthetic when I went back to work three days later. Over the years it had never ceased to amaze me how easily people succumbed to sickness, or took the odd "duvet" day.

Yet on that particular evening I understood why people had weeks off with stress, so I gave myself a good talking too, and regained my positive attitude that thankfully it did not desert me again.

There had been an incident that had happened to someone close to me in another trust that made me think about the organisation for which I worked. The incident led to suspension, and came close to the loss of Registration to Practice. The manager concerned, and equally at fault, as she did not support her DNS when she should have done, got off scot-free. This heavy handed and unjust approach still makes me seethe when I think about it, and ashamed that people are not bought to account when they should be in the age of so called transparency.

In my line of work I had come across people who had not been able to achieve their hopes and dreams of retirement. In their working years they would plan to go travelling, or take up a hobby or sport. Then fate stepped in, and soon after the much coveted day of retirement one of the couple had a major health crisis. Elsie and Ken had sold up to buy a place in Spain, and were at least able to enjoy it for a year, until Ken had a stroke. When I met them as a DN, they were trying to cope in a mobile home. Ken, a big man needed a hospital bed, ceiling track hoist, riser recliner armchair, and wheelchair. Manoeuvring him in the tiny space available, was very difficult, especially for his carers who did his personal care, and the DNs who visited. This awful situation continued for years until Ken died, and Elsie went into a home with dementia.

Alan and Sheila had a daughter who had aggressive multiple sclerosis, and their time was fully taken up with her well being, as their trips to France faded into the distance. Their daughter was very angry about her illness, and her parents fought her corner, and managed to get her a purpose built flat for disability, which Kate, as a designer had decorated beautifully. When Kate died, I did not see her parents until I took Alan on to my CM caseload years later.

Alan had gradually gone downhill with heart disease and dementia. He started wandering from the house, early one morning before Sheila woke, he took himself up to the shops. Luckily the butchers were in their shop around six am, realised something was amiss, popped Alan in the car and delivered him to the local residential home for the elderly. The staff at the home took him in, made him comfortable with a cup of tea, found identification on him, and phoned his wife. Sheila had quite a scare as she had not realised he was missing. Soon after he went to a nursing home as his wife could no longer manage him at home. The decision was very hard for Sheila, especially as Alan did not settle in his new home, thought he was being attacked, and barricaded his room so the staff couldn't get in. I thought of Alan when I first knew him, and contemplated what a poor hand of life had been dealt to him and his family.

Despite fate that changed a retirees plan, others coped, and relished in what could of been, realised it would be impossible to achieve, and settled for something they could enjoy. In patients with a chronic condition, with gradual deterioration over about fifteen years before death, compromise meant they had a reasonable quality of life, and learnt to utilise the good days, and rest on the bad days. Nita with chronic heart failure loved to play bingo, if she felt well she went, and if not she stayed at home. Mum and Pops in Law had years of happy retirement with long trips on their narrow boat, travelled abroad and enjoyed it all. They had lost their daughter to leukaemia in her childhood, and despite this Mum used to say: "What ever happens we have had a good life", and I thought I want to be able to say that too, and so far I could. Like my in laws, Alistair and I had been on several far destination holidays, and planned to go again later in life, but in case we couldn't at least we had been once. Unlike my patients that had left all their aspirations until they retired, and then had their dreams snatched away, due to ill health of themselves, partner or family member.

When I attended work meetings I had long since developed the art of not allowing them to eat into my clinical or home time. At the start I would state to the chair person that I was conscious of time, and would have to leave on the dot at the end of the meeting. If it ended at four, I would get up, thank the chair, and go regardless of progress, as I felt a well ordered meeting should not overrun. Nine times out of ten the important work had been covered, and we had entered what I called the aimless banter stage. This was when everyone put in their little bit, or when asked if anything else needed to be said, everyone would be quiet, except one, that led to a further half hour or more with no useful outcome.

We all gathered in the Seminar Room at Bath Road, for a meeting one afternoon, and our Head of Adult Services asked everyone where we thought we would be in five years time? Quick as a flash, and without thinking about it, I promptly responded "retired". The HAS paused, smiled, acknowledged the idea, and asked apart from retirement, how we saw the Trust in five years time. It became "time to smile and wave", a technique I had developed for meetings, adopted from the animated film Penguin. Each time visitors came, the penguins would show them what they wanted to see, and everyone went home happy.

In early 2013 we were mulling over the day's events in the bath one evening, and Alistair looked at me, and said: "Let's retire". This really took the bull by the horns. But what were we doing? Both working full time, to have ever increased work demands in the name of autonomy. In our mid fifties, our original employment pension schemes allowed retirement at fifty five, we did not need to go on to sixty or sixty five. Charlie and Vikki were happily married in their first house, and Georgette and Duncan, engaged and making plans for their wedding. I had already attended the Pre Retirement session at work twice, and went a third time. There was a great deal of useful information, and I wanted to make sure I had everything clear. We talked to as many retirees as possible, to find out what they lived on. The Moneyadvice online budget tool enabled us to objectively assess monthly income and expenditure in retirement. Both of us could claim occupational pensions, and a lump sun. We concluded if we rented the house out to supplement income, and bought a motorhome to tour and live in, finance would be sufficient.

With protracted thought we drafted a letter of resignation to our employers, then, I got cold feet, the end of October four months away was too soon for me. I still loved and enjoyed the clinical side of my work, and I knew in my mind, once I resigned I could not go back to nursing. The steady tide of change that I kept pace with, would accelerate away, and for me be impossible to regain. The other factor was, I wanted to ensure the trust had interviewed and offered my post to a new CM before I left, so I could meet her and give a proper hand over of my patients. In view of this Alistair and I re-drafted and submitted our resignation for the end of March the following year, it panned out to be the right decision, and I began to look forward and plan for a life without work.

There proved much preparation to do. At home I did

not have the heart to through out all my academic professional work, and neither did I want to store it. Early one morning I sealed all the folders up in a box with my name on it. Then, at my base I buried the box deep in a cupboard that was always a tip, and never tidied by those responsible. My hidden box will probably remain there for years, ready for me if I should ever need it. I carefully reviewed my patients to make sure everything was up to date and in order. I decided to tell them of my retirement well in advance of the date, and prepare them for the change. This proved to be the most difficult part, as many relied on me entirely for health guidance, and had benefited from the time invested in them.

My replacement had been appointed, and I met up with her to hand over my patients, and explain the complex working of the job, and the many little useful foibles that helped the job run smoothly. There would be a short gap as the new CM worked her notice in the heart failure team, so I introduced my colleague CM to my patients, who agreed to oversee in the meantime, and be on the end of the phone for them. For my patients to have my direct number had been one of the most valued aspects of the service.

For the last visit for each of my patients I allowed plenty of time, accepted a cup of tea for once, and after the health requirements were completed we sat and chatted. I think this really helped them and me say goodbye to each other, and our parting of the ways. Many of them gave me momentous, these will always remind me of that person, and my fascinating role as CM, and to look back fondly on my nursing career.

I can hear my colleagues in the main hall prepare for the retirement lunch, that Alison and I will share. After a working lifetime as a nurse Alison has also decided to resign her team leader post, and retire. Twelve o'clock has come, and I sign off my laptop for the last time, and join all my colleagues. There is a super spread, as is customary everyone has supplied a dish, along with a homemade cake complete with stethoscope and syringe icing. My CM colleague does the introductory speech, then my team leader and nurse manager, who I have known throughout my community career thank us both for our commitment and hard work over the years, adding in a few funny moments, that make everyone laugh. Senior management send congratulations, as they have an important meeting and are unable to come, although Alison and I have accumulated nearly eighty years service between us. We both have wonderful flowers and gifts. The trust thoughtfully gave me a voucher, that amounted to the equivalent of two pounds seventy seven pence per year of service. My NM checked my equipment, and that I would drop my uniform in, and that was it. Freedom and the Seven Day Weekend!

Epilogue

Alistair and I retired on the last day of March 2014, gave ourselves a month to rent our house out, and buy a motorhome to tour and live in full time. Our Burstner 875 IXEO Plus is our current home. A year since retirement we have spent eight months touring France, Spain and Portugal, and are now back in the UK seeing friends and family. In September 2015, we plan to be off again, to further satisfy our curiosity and wanderlust, and fulfil more of our dreams.

Glossary of Terms

Anaemia. Various causes, e.g. low iron levels.

Anti-epileptics. Drugs that control epilepsy.

Asepsis. Sterile procedure and area.

Atrial fibrillation Irregularity in heart beat.

Aventis. Drug manufacturer.

Back trolley. Colloquial name for ward equipment trolley.

Baise. Green non stretch support for Thomas splint.

Barn Door. Abnormal ECG showing myocardial infarct.

Base line observations. Temp pulse blood pressure O2 saturation.

Bayer. Drug manufacturer.

Bean counter. Slang for accountants.

BHSAI. British Horse Society Assistant Instructor.

Bite Size. Training for community matrons.

Blood glucose. Blood sugar.

Boots. Drug manufacturer.

Bronchioles. Part of lung.

Burr Hole. Drilling through scull to relieve pressure.

Cachexic. Extreme weight loss in terminal cancer.

Calcaneus. Heel bone.

Cannula. Used for giving fluid or taking blood.

CAS. Continence Advisory Service.

Carpel tunnel. Wrist operation.

CC. Case Coordinator.

Cerebral embolus. Blood clot in the brain.

Cervix. Neck of uterus.

CHNE. Community Health Nurse for the Elderly.

Clubbing. Shape of fingers after prolonged chest conditions.

CM. Community Matron.

Commissioning. Buying services from other Provider health departments.

CNS. Community Nursing Sister (without DN qualification).

Co-codamol Pain relief, codeine phosphate and paracetamol.

Controlled drugs. Narcotic drugs.

QOF. Quality Outcomes Framework.

COPD. Chronic obstructive pulmonary disease.

CPT. Community Practice Teacher.

CQC. Care Quality Commission.

CQUIN. Commissioning for Quality and Innovation.

Crash Trolley. Emergency resuscitation trolley.

CSSD. Central Sterile Supply Department.

CV. Curriculum vitae.

Diuretic. Medication to reduce water retention in body.

DNS. District Nursing Sister.

DN. District Nurse.

DOH. Department of Health.

Doppler Ultrasound. Machine to assess circulation in the legs.

DVT Deep Vein Thrombosis. a blood clot in the leg.

ECT. Electro Convulsive Therapy.

ECG. Electrocardiogram.

ENB. English National Board.

Entonox. Inhaled analgesia for pain control.

ERS. Electronic Record System.

Essence of Care. Government initiative to improve care.

EUSOL. Exeter University Solution of Lime.

Flatus. Wind from bowel.

Four layer. Elasticated bandage system.

Fructosamine. Measurement of blood glucose over last three months.

Fund Holding. Replaced by, and similar to Commissioning.

GP. General Practitioner.

G-strap. Prevents pulling of urinary catheter.

Glucometer Home monitoring device for blood glucose.

HA. Health Authority.

HAS. Head of Adult Services.

HBAIC. HaemoglobinAIC Measurement of blood glucose over last six weeks.

HCA. Health Care Assistant.

Hidradenitis suppurativa. A condition where boils form over lymph glands.

HV. Health Visitor.

Hyperglycaemia. High blood glucose.

Hypoglycaemia. Low blood glucose.

Hyponatremia. Low sodium in blood.

Hypoxia. Low oxygen level.

ICU. Intensive Care Unit.

Infalog. Hand held unit for data collection.

Ipratropium (Atrovent), bronchodilator, keeps airways open.

Jelonet. Paraffin coated gauze dressing.

Kaltostat. A wound dressing derived from seaweed.

Ketones. Inadvertent breakdown of fat and protein for energy.

LDT. Learning Disabilities Team.

Matron. Senior nurse position above Sister.

Medical Loans. Original equipment loans service.

Mepitel. Modern silicon dressing.

MDT. Multi Disciplinary Team.

Myocardial Infarct. Heart attack.

NA. Nursing Auxiliary.

Nasal Cannula. Oxygen delivery via the nose.

Nasogastric tube. Inserted through the nose to the stomach.

Nebuliser.Machine to administer inhaled medication.

Necrotic. Black dead tissue.

Nelson's Inhaler. An inhalation of Friars Balsam.

Nephropathy. Damage to kidneys.

Neuropathy. Damage to nerves.

NH. Nursing Home.

Nightingale Ward. Layout of ward designed by Florence Nightingale.

NM. Nurse Manager (previously Neighbourhood Manager).

No7. Senior nurse position (now and before Matron).

NRS Berkshire Equipment Services. Trust loans service.

O2. Oxygen.

O2 saturation. Level of O2 in blood.

Oedematous. Fluid filled.

Oesophageal Irrigation Secret code for a cup of tea/ coffee etc.

OLDCART. Onset, Location, Duration, Aggravators, Relievers, Treatment.

Oncology. Study of cancer.

Otoscope. Instrument for ear examination.

Oral hypoglycaemics. Group of drugs to lower blood glucose.

PDP. Professional Development Plan.

Paracetamol (Panadol) pain relief.

PQRST. Markers used in ECG reading.

Prednisolone. Steroid.

Provider. Health services for Commissioners to buy.

Pulmonary embolus. Blood clot in lungs.

Pulse oximeter. Small instrument to assess oxygen levels.

Pursed lip breathing. Oxygen conservation technique.

Rapid Response Team. Urgent care to prevent hospital admission.

RBH. Royal Berkshire Hospital.

RGN. Registered General Nurse.

Redivac drain. Vacuumed drain for operation site.

Retinopathy. Damage to retina of eye.

RISK. Computer program to identify high risk patients.

Rivaroxaban. Anticoagulant.

Roho cushion/ heel boots. Low air skin pressure relief.

Salbutamol (Ventolin). short acting bronchodilator.

Seretide. Long acting bronchodilator, steroid.

SEN. State Enrolled Nurse.

Short stretch. Two layer bandage system.

Slough. Dead grey tissue.

SMINT. Self Managed Integrated Nursing Team.

SN. Staff Nurse.

Sofban. Synthetic wool bandage..

Spirometer. Machine to assess lung function.

Spirometry. Lung function test.

Spooning. Shape of nails in chronic chest condition.

SRN. State Registered Nurse.

Sphygmanomete.r Machine to measure blood pressure.

Sporran bag/ belt Urinary drainage system.

StN / St Nurse. Student Nurse.

Supra pubic catheter. For urine drainage via abdomen.

Surgipad. Secondary absorbent wound dressing.

Swan-neck. Part of traction for Thomas splint.

Terminal Cancer. Incurable cancer close to death.

The Six Cs. Government initiative to improve nursing care.

Tiotropium. long acting anticholenergic bronchodilator.

Three way pulley Part of traction for Thomas splint.

Thomas splint. Support splint used for fractured femur (thigh bone).

Tracheotomy. Incision in neck for breathing.

Trachy/ tracheostomy tube. Metal or plastic to facilitate breathing.

Trocanter. Anatomical part of thigh bone (femur).

Urea and electrolytes. Substances in blood used for monitoring a condition.

Urethra. Anatomical tube from bladder to urethral meatus.

Urethral meatus. Exit of urethra to outside body.

Urinary catheter. Tube inserted into the bladder for urine drainage.

Vacutainer. Holds needle and bottle during venepuncture.

Venepuncture.Taking blood.

William and Marrow. W and M both abnormal ECG patterns.

Warfarin. Anticoagulant.

www.ingramcontent.com/pod-product-compliance
Lightning Source LLC
Chambersburg PA
CBHW051902170526
45168CB00001B/204